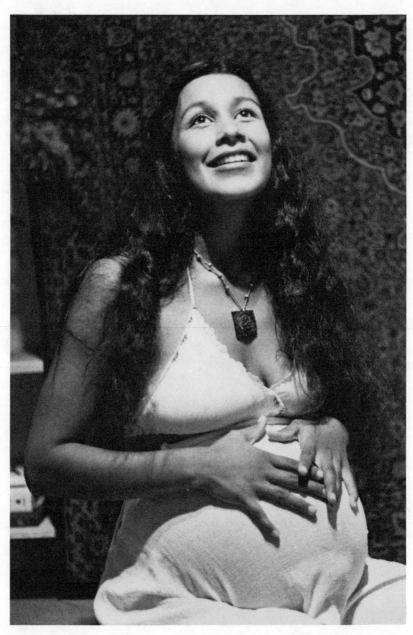

TRANSFORMATION THROUGH BIRTH

TRANSFORMATION THROUGH BIRTH

A Woman's Guide

Claudia Panuthos

Foreword by Suzanne Arms

Bergin & Garvey Publishers, Inc.
Massachusetts

Library of Congress Cataloging and Publication Data

Panuthos, Claudia.
  Transformation through birth.

  Bibliography: p. 181
  Includes index.
  1. Pregnancy.   2. Childbirth.   I. Title.
RG525.P245 1983   618.2′4   83-15559
ISBN 0-89789-037-X
ISBN 0-89789-038-8 (pbk.)

Published in 1984 by Bergin & Garvey Publishers, Inc.
670 Amherst Road
South Hadley, Massachusetts 01075

Printed in the United States of America

987654321

Cover design by Patricia Greene
Cover photo © Suzanne Arms

Contents

Foreword

Childbirth is a good metaphor for life. It has its time of conception, then long gestation followed by hard labor to bring forth a new creation. There is passion and often pain before fulfillment. The way we birth has always been greatly affected by our culture. When a society is in turmoil, and unconsciousness prevails, childbirth, too, reflects turmoil and unconsciousness.

For every person going through the process of birth, there is the possibility of transformation at the individual and the family level. That is why so many of us view birth as such a critical time, a hopeful time. In another decade or two we may look back upon the women giving birth today and feel grateful that an entire generation worked so hard to enable their sisters and their daughters to have the benefit of a transformed consciousness in birth.

In many ways, birth has become the crucible in which modern woman is ground and burned: it is our testing place. But there is value in this work. Now, as in no other time I know of,women have the capacity to break through what binds us and keeps us crippled and dependent in birth. True—our births have often been difficult and painful, but pain can be an essential part of growth. We can choose to birth consciously and to face what labor brings us. We are freeing ourselves from a centuries-old legacy of fear. Perhaps that is why it is not easy, and why so often our births have not matched our ideals. Unfortunately this gap between possibility and reality has left many of us with guilt, self-recrimination, resentment, and rage.

Anger has been a part of our healing. But anger seldom does us personal good, whether it is suppressed or directed at others. There has been much to rage against —injustice, cruelty, a patriarchal system, insensitive institutions and unyielding professionals. The time for using our energy in justifiable rage is passing. A different voice is required of us now, especially if we are actively working toward a non-violent world.

This book is a guide for these difficult times, a companion any woman can take on her journey. We need such a companion. No matter how good we feel about our growth and our accomplishments in the outer world over the past few years, birth is a different story. Birth requires a more receptive, yielding kind of creativity — something few of us know much about. Birth is still our Achilles' heel, the place where we can easily be reduced to terror and dependency. We have not yet stopped long enough to turn inward and heal the hurts that history imposed on us through our reproduction. As long as we fear being taken over by a process that is bigger than we are and which is outside our mind's control, as birth is; and so long as we continue to place ourselves in the care of people who do not fully understand or support us or trust this process, then we are left weak at our core, in our most creative, procreative place.

Today most books on preparation for childbirth focus on adding more information rather than helping to affirm our inner knowledge; on *doing* rather than *being*. Most books are full of How-To advice, as if we would birth more confidently and easily if only we knew *more* and tried *harder*. The real task is in being able to live what we can envision. And even for many women who, like myself, will never birth again, the task is to heal scars that are still infecting our lives and our relationships. As Claudia Panuthos points out so well, today our work lies mainly in self-acceptance.

This book offers wisdom into the processes of the psyche—wisdom acquired through the human potential movement. It provides a vision of birth, relationship, and life that is whole and life-affirming, without denying pain and hard work. It gives insights which can help us lay a new foundation for a transformative experience through birth, which is what birth *can* be. It offers special support for men and for their unique burdens. It is written by a woman whose words resonate with understanding of the problems, and compassion for everyone. Claudia Panuthos knows what she is talking about, drawing not only from her own experience of giving birth, but also from observing the hundreds of women who have attended her workshops and have been counseled for problems associated with childbirth. By finding ways to help women who are scarred by traumatic births heal themselves, Claudia has found what can help *every* woman.

This is a feminist book in the fullest sense of the word because it is a guide to enabling and releasing our potential. It underscores the special capacity human beings have for reshaping the past and for transforming the present through a new consciousness. It does more for the growth of women than any book on birth I've read in years. In reading it, I felt a lightening up and a releasing of emotions still left from my own birth, and from the birth of my daughter thirteen years ago. I have done a lot to free myself from the past. This has been one more step.

Suzanne Arms
Portola Valley, California

Preface

Kahlil Griban once wrote, "Show me your mother's face: I'll tell you who you are." He was referring to the profound significance of the maternal-child relationship, a relationship he believed was built on the boundless, relentless love of a mother for her offspring. This relationship begins long before birth and is manifested in the childbirth experience. Childbearing, because of its awesome emotional impact, is often the basis of family relationship patterns and parental self-images for many years to follow.

Thousands and perhaps millions of women throughout the United States begin the experience of motherhood feeling guilty and inadequate over the events of pregnancy and birth. Most suffer silently the hurt resulting from medicated or surgical deliveries, from unwanted (and in some cases, unneeded) hospital interventions, from pregnancy related losses and countless unmet needs.

Today's childbearing woman attempts to give birth in a political atmosphere of conflict, confusion and change. As modern day obstetrical practices are challenged, the childbearing woman becomes increasingly pressured (both externally and internally) to birth correctly and even perfectly. In 1979 *The People Place,* a family counseling service, began a specialized program for child-bearing parents seeking relief and release from these pressures.

Over the past four years, we have worked with thousands of women seeking emotional release and psychological resolutions to pregnancy and childbirth conflicts and violations. Hundreds of phone calls and letters have come to us from women throughout this country and Canada representing a wide span in ages, backgrounds and geographic locations. Each of these women express a uniquely different but equally important need for not only resolution but also adequate psychological preparation. In attempting to meet the hundreds of requests for a psychological approach to these issues, a new counseling center called *Offspring* opened its door in the fall of 1982.

Transformation Through Birth was written to provide childbearing men and women with a sound psychological approach to resolving the past and preparing for positive future experiences. It draws upon many years of clinical experience as a family therapist as well as personal experiences as a childbearing woman and mother and is offered to the thousands, perhaps millions, of parents who might otherwise begin family life in conflict and stress.

No childbirth education course is adequate without a psychological base. No childbearing woman is prepared to give birth unless she has sought personal understanding of the emotional and psychological impact that becoming a parent often brings. The concepts and tools presented in this material are designed to aid childbearing parents in such understanding and preparation.

Transformation Through Birth offers parents the techniques of mind-body integration and the opportunity for adequate and realistic emotional preparation for childbirth with an approach that supports the healthy, positive outcomes we all naturally desire. This book is dedicated to the idea that maternal well-being *positive birthing* and healthy integration are of paramount importance to us all. Perhaps one day we, as childbearing women, will truly celebrate the physical magnificence of our bodies without grading our shapes; the inborn capacity to bear and to love our children without demanding perfection; and the innate worth of our own existence without performing for approval.

Claudia Panuthos
OFFSPRING
Arlington, Massachusetts

Acknowledgements

to

Nancy Brown   *Patricia Flagg*
Diane Koster   *Paul Guyton*
Elaine Bontempo   *John Miller*
Lee Longchamps   *Peter Panuthos*
Catherine Romeo   *Jonathan Panuthos*
Nancy Wainer Cohen   *Kim Cavanaugh*

and to all the women and men who have so willingly shared their stories.

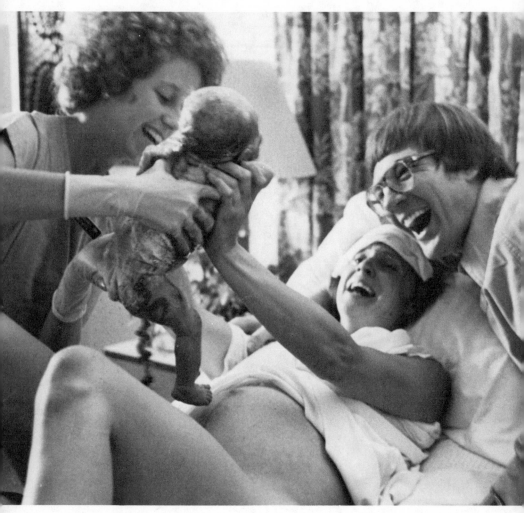

1

Positive Birthing:
A Definition

Birth is the beginning; the beginning of life, of parenthood, of family. It is the foundation and groundwork for future family functioning. It is the initial contact between infants and parents, and a welcoming celebration of a new life into the world.

Every family deserves a positive beginning and every parent and child an emotionally conscious birthing. Positive birthing is an approach to childbirth that emphasizes the internal experience of each man and woman and the effect of that internal experience on the parent, spouse, child, and entire family system. It does not include any specific technique, intervention, exercise, environment, or outcome, all of which can be very important. Rather, it is an approach designed to free parents from the nightmarish legacy of guilt and self-disapproval common to Western childbearing practices and fueled by present pressures to birth perfectly.

There is much social pressure today to birth our children in the "right" way, in the "right" place, and with all the "right" people. It is certainly true that creating a supportive birth team, becoming an informed consumer, and actively choosing how and where to birth are all supportive of positive birthing. However, when giving birth at home, breathing correctly, following Leboyer's (1974) plan for a gentle birth, or getting the right set of photographs supersedes the psychological well-being of women, the entire family system suffers greatly—and perhaps permanently. So, the first and primary focus of positive birthing is the psychological, physical, and spiritual well-being of childbearing women.

Psychological Obstacles to Well-Being

Psychological health is the connecting force to physical, emotional, and spiritual well-being. Books as old as the Bible remind us, "What we sow in the mind, we reap in the body," and "What a man [or woman] thinketh, so he [or she] is." With total well-being as a primary goal, prenatal nutrition, psychological preparation for labor and childbirth, and emotional adjustment to family life can become opportunities for personal growth. For example, it is well known to most psychotherapists that there is great difficulty involved in assisting an overweight client with dieting or an anorexic teenager with eating, when he or she is depressed or lacking in confidence and a sense of self-worth. Gail Brewer, in her book *What Every Pregnant Woman Should Know* (1977), describes the necessity of good prenatal nutrition and its effect on the childbearing process. Phyllis Williams's work *Nourishing Your Unborn Child* (1974) resounds with support for adequate and healthful nourishment during pregnancy. Yet, if the psychological state of a childbearing woman is one of self-ridicule, perfectionistic demands, isolation, or internalized societal pressures, it will be unlikely that an expectant mother will be able to follow these programs with genuine consistency or heartfelt self-support.

Healthy Mind Yields Healthy Body

Although, with the current return to midwifery and care by nurse practitioners, women are receiving better nutritional information and follow-up, they are often unable to give it effect in a daily diet. One midwife recently shared her frustration in trying to get a young pregnant woman to eat adequately and avoid potential anemia. The woman, mother of a 3-year-old child, was alone most of the day, depressed at the prognosis of a future of more isolated mothering, and anxious not to break her commitment to a vegetarian diet. After some simple changes were made geared toward improving the woman's psychological condition (a regular baby-sitter, a women's support group, etc.), she began to eat more often and in larger quantities. She was then able to improve her iron count so dramatically that she could qualify for the home birth she desired, while still adhering to her vegetarian diet.

Women who fear weight gain (supported by the well-meant but sometimes harmful obstetrical practice of creating anxiety in women who gain more than 25 pounds) often eat inadequately. Although the Society for the Protection of the Unborn through Nutrition (SPUN) reports that 30,000 infants die needlessly and that 200,000 children with preventable birth defects are born each year, because of prematurity and low birth weights (Kenefick

1981), the American woman's psychological well-being is so often connected to thinness that fear of fat is actually killing children.

SPUN reports remind us that babies with the lowest incidence of brain damage are born to mothers who gain 36 pounds or more during pregnancy (Kenefick 1981). Some possible 200,000 babies suffer preventable birth defects because we have failed to free ourselves of the false sense of inner well-being achieved through a thin body.

"Stress," not "Distress"

The primary goal of well-being also supports the emotional stability necessary for the normal stress of labor. Gayle Peterson describes birth as stress, but reminds us that it is also a normal, natural condition of childbirth. It is only when stress is ignored or denied that its effects may become damaging and manifest as mental unrest or physical disease. As Peterson writes, "Hopefully it does not become distress" (Peterson 1981).

A woman who is adequately prepared for the reality of labor and delivery, and who has mobilized her psychological resources in advance, is far more likely to achieve the natural childbirth so many couples prepare for. She may not achieve ecstasy, but will, perhaps, be more attuned to the realities of childbearing and to herself.

Postpartum Blues: Not Necessary

If all our systems, both internal and external, were truly dedicated to maternal well-being, women would be far less likely to suffer prolonged postpartum blues. Most studies indicate that some postpartum depression is a normal condition in Western women. Hamburg et al. (1968) found that two-thirds of a group of postpartum mothers they studied cried for trivial reasons—a condition they described as unusual. It is true that postnatal depression and grieving are normal states (also health states, as I hope to show later in this work). Psychologically fit women are far more likely to pass through this healing process effectively and return quickly to a state of integrated family life.

Mental-health statistics indicate that the American woman of childbearing age is the most likely candidate for psychiatric hospital admission for depressive disorders than anyone else in the population. Further, approximately 4,000 postpartum women are hospitalized for psychiatric disorders annually (U.S. Department of Mental Health Reports 1981). Perhaps with a dedication to psychological well-being at the time of pregnancy and childbearing (a time of great emotional stress), we can avoid the painful effects of long-term unconsciousness and denial of women's needs so common to the American mother.

What Is "Positive Birthing"?

Positive birthing is a psychophysiological (mind-body) approach to child birth that focuses on the harmonious integration of body, mind, heart, and soul. The mind and body, when aligned, dance in rhythm and unity, surrendering willingly to the new life coming forth. Most women and men are learning much-needed physiological information in preparation for childbirth, information that is extremely necessary for positive birthing and informed consumerism. There is, however, the additional component of psychological preparation and understanding that supports the physiological process. Positive birthing is an approach to physical birthing based on sound psychological principles.

Suzanne Arms, in *Immaculate Deception* (1975), writes, "For all the talk, the popularity, the trendiness and occasional faddishness surrounding natural childbirth, the process itself is seldom achieved." Nancy Cohen and Lois Estner, in *Silent Knife* (1983), reveal some alarming statistics that indicate a Cesarean delivery rate of 17 to 20 percent—over 30 percent in many hospitals—and an episiotomy rate of 90 percent. Only about 10 percent of the 3.5 million American women giving birth each year do so naturally. It is hoped that a sound psychological basis will increase the chances for childbearing experiences with minimal intervention that are based on an informed choice as well as on psychological well-being. In this framework, women can be emotionally as well as physically conscious and learn to rely on their own inner resources as well as on sound medical advice.

"Natural" Childbirth: A Qualified "Yes"

Studies on the use of drugs in labor and delivery indicate a potential danger to both mother and child. In addition, studies of women who actively participate in childbirth seem to indicate great gains in personal resources and self-confidence through the experience of childbirth. Although natural childbirth is not synonymous in any way with positive birthing, it is certainly a goal supportive of maternal and infant well-being and therefore will be discussed in terms of psychophysiology.

"Painless" Childbirth: An Unfortunate Myth

Fernand Lamaze (1958) developed a concept of "painless" childbirth out of his observations of Russian obstetrics in the 1950s and his understanding of the effects of mental conditioning on somatic manifestations. He set in motion a process for returning to Western women a much-needed sense of control over childbearing based on disciplined breathing. He helped to take some of the drama out of labor and some of the drugs out of childbirth.

Unfortunately, his work became the basis for a misleading notion that childbirth can be painless. Obviously, no one wants to be in pain. In fact, it is our pain-avoidance reflex that prevents us from injuring ourselves, for example, on a hot stove or a sharp tool. Pain, in labor and birth, is an unwanted reality, but a vastly different pain than one would incur from the hot stove or sharp tool. Childbirth educators who attempt to discuss the reality of pain have often shared at seminars their own frustration at communicating the reality of pain to an audience that spaces out and seems to go unconscious in the discussion. The very healthy pain-avoidance reflex does not even want to talk about pain and accepts misleading illusions of painless birth.

The Lamaze techniques provided women with a role in childbearing and a disciplined breathing technique that have been both a blessing and a curse. The blessing for us all is that we as women were given the support we needed to find out that we can, in fact, give birth out of our own resources. The curse is in the idea of control rather than surrender, and discipline rather than release. The psychophysiological necessity for surrender and release will be discussed throughout this material so that all breathing techniques can lead to mental peace rather than tension and control.

Voices of Postpartum Women

Dr. Lamaze (1958) categorized the births of several thousand women. His category called "failure" were those women who experienced restlessness and who screamed. We know now that although wild, unfocused screaming causes women to lose force that is needed for labor and delivery, focused and integrated emotional expression can greatly aid in the surrender and release necessary for giving birth. Many Lamaze "failures" who screamed were expressing the natural life-giving forces of birth. Women from all over the United States and Canada have shared their support. Some 82 percent of our files of hundreds of letters were written by women angered by the childbirth preparation teaching they received; these women expressed their need to yell out in joy, hurt, pain, fear, and life at the time of their children's births. Some of their post-birth evaluations of disciplined breathing are as follows:

> *I believed my instructor when she said childbirth could be painless. Imagine my surprise! [Carolyn—New York.]*
> *I took classes and practiced breathing. I did everything exactly as I was taught. There must be another way [Rose—New Hampshire].*
> *Thanks so much for saying in our seminar that the usual breathing for control and discipline doesn't work. I was feeling like such a failure. I felt like I was running from my baby by focusing away [Alison—Connecticut].*

The misleading notion that childbirth can be painless has caused deep feelings of failure in those women who did not have "painless" births. They blame themselves for not exercising enough, for not breathing properly, and for being too weak-minded to dismiss the pain. Even the adaptations of the Lamaze system have only sent more couples huffing, puffing, and panting their way into exhaustion and despair. It *is*, however, possible to reach a state free of pain. Ina May Gaskin's findings and stories from *Spiritual Midwifery* (1977) indicate a switch in the contractions from pain to "energy rushes," where pain is transformed into a higher consciousness, in much the way described for Eastern meditative disciplines. These conditions are not achieved by focusing concentration away from pain. As Suzanne Arms (1975) comments about the Lamaze technique, "It has the unfortunate side effect of greatly altering a woman's natural experience of birth from one of deep involvement inside of her body to a controlled distraction." Gayle Peterson (1981) supports this view in her instructions for breathing focus in labor, constantly directing a woman to her own "inner breath" and encouraging women toward "inner focus." Techniques based on avoidance of pain, fear, or loss of control only lead to pain, fear, and loss of control, as the psychological resistance attracts what it repels.

Childbirth "without Fear": Another Progressive Illusion

Around the same time that Lamaze developed the notion of painless childbirth, Grantly Dick-Read developed the idea of "childbirth without fear," the title of his work (Dick-Read 1944). Again, Dick-Read's contributions were significant to the state of obstetrical practices at the time, since he was essentially the first to notice environmental conditions as a source of tension and fear. He developed the idea that natural childbirth enables a woman to feel a greater sense of control and thus reduces fear, which produces physical tension. The ultimate manifestation was observed in the fear-tension-pain response that resulted in ineffective labor and white uterus (a condition where the uterus lacks red blood cells necessary for contracting).

The idea of natural childbirth has greatly aided women in retrieving a sense of control over childbirth and paved the way for a husband-supported model such as that developed by Bradley, author of *Husband Coached Childbirth* (1965). Understanding the need for anxiety-reducing environments and psychological support has further improved our birthing practices. Again, however, this approach has led to a second misleading notion: that of childbirth without fear. Dick-Read's approach to lessening fear through education was soundly based, in that information tends to quiet the mind. However, the mind also fills in any unknown future outcome with a continuous flow of potential negative possibilities such as a difficult labor, a deformed child, or a generally upsetting birth. These fears are natural and normal and usually pass like clouds on a windy day when left without any accompanying intense emotional impact. The idea of "childbirth without fear" is an illusion that has led women to believe they were at best over-anxious mothers and at worst hysterical personalities. Fear is a psychic necessity that is the precursor for situational evaluation of certain conditions. Many women are enabled to refuse internal fetal monitors, drugs, enemas, and shavings by their fear that their children will suffer if they accept these procedures.

Recognizing and understanding the nature of fear is far more likely to yield the positive outcomes we all desire. Although cognitive data may quiet mental questions resulting from unknown possibilities, childbirth without fear is an impossible illusion.

Avoidance Breeds Pain

Avoiding anything becomes resistance. For example, most experts on pain know that relaxation and surrender reduce pain. Resistance increases pain. Resistance, even through disciplined breathing, then becomes counter-productive and in some cases actually increases pain. As Sheila Kitzinger (1981) says, "If a woman tries to resist or even endure contractions, she will have severe pain. She must go with them and cooperate with them in getting her baby born." This is also true of hospital politics. If a labor coach is more interested in resisting hospital policies or physicians' interventions, the birthing woman is more likely to incur unnecessary interference and vio-lations, since the psychological battle incites the physician to prove his way correct. This does not mean that labor coaches should not seek the best for birthing women or that unnecessary obstetrical practices should continue. It does mean that any resistance to these conditions will result in their increased manifestation rather than their reduction. It means that adequate psychological preparation for pain and adequate knowledge and understand-ing of fear are far more likely to produce positive birthings.

Inner Attitudes the Core of Positive Birthing

William James (1950) wrote, "The greatest discovery in our generation is that human beings, by changing the inner attitudes of their minds, can change the outer aspects of their lives." The effects of mental beliefs on psychological functioning, along with techniques for releasing past beliefs and establishing positive mental systems, will be discussed in the chapters ahead. It is impossible to know every personal thought or belief about birth. However, we owe ourselves the opportunity for as much mental conscious-ness and awareness as possible. The chapters ahead will provide the op-portunity to examine individual beliefs and perhaps to alter those that do not support positive birthing and maternal well-being. Once altered, the mind can develop loving thoughts and supportive beliefs that affirm maternal health, confidence, and faith in the innate ability of the human body to birth naturally.

Healthy Integration: The Essential Process

Finally, positive birthing is an approach built on the important principle that healthy psychological integration is of paramount importance. Regardless of external events, we all need peace of mind. "Integration" is defined in *Taber's Cyclopedic Medical Dictionary* (1970) as "assimilation; a harmonious relationship of the parts constituting the whole of anything." Samuels and Bennett, in *Be Well* (1974), developed a scale measurement of ease and disease ranging from 1 through 12, with 1 representing joy (ease) and 12 representing pain and suffering (disease). In their system, the key to understanding one's own sense of ease and disease, and maintaining personal well-being, lies in trusting one's own feelings, which provide "an intimate link between inborn healing abilities and self-regulating processes."

Healthy Integration: A Definition

Healthy integration of childbirth experiences, then, refers to a harmonious relationship of all birthing events that yield "ease" and peace of mind. Any feelings that do not reflect harmony and unity yield discomfort, pain, and suffering, and perhaps dis-ease. Parents deserve to remain emotionally conscious on childbearing events in order to fully engage all inborn healing abilities and to integrate, to assimilate, all birth-related events with health and peace.

Realistic Visions

In order to accomplish healthy integration, it is useful to begin with realistic visions. Unfortunately, fairy-tale approaches to childbirth without fear, pain, or reality burden the mind with idealistic mental pictures of ecstasy and discount the human reality of occasional agony. The picture-perfect birth scenes where everything goes as planned usually lead to some sense of disappointment and failure. Couples desperately trying to maintain control are far more likely to lose it.

We are living in a quick-fix, get-high, feel-good culture. We have come to view anything that causes upset as bad and therefore to be avoided. We have failed to see that great resources are built out of managing stress and that much personal growth often results. Labor is not easy or quick. It is not without pain for most women. In fact, it is tedious and exhausting. Pushing a baby out is not effortless, but it is effort worthwhile. Birth is agony and ecstasy. Life is agony and ecstasy. Hopefully, we learn from the agony and bask in the ecstasy.

Releasing Negative Emotions

For some, healthy integration may mean a release of hurt, anger, disappointment, guilt, sorrow, or inadequacy related to the events of childbirth. Most theories of Western psychotherapy (for example, Gestalt, bioenergetics, and primal therapy) are built on the principle of release of emotionally charged upsets in order to find peace of mind and health of body. Virginia Satir (1978) wrote that most of us live in emotional jails guarded by our own inner demands for obedience, goodness, and rightness. The chapters ahead are an invitation to all childbearing couples who suffer inner pain to break out of the emotional jails and release birth-related hurts whenever possible. There are several suggestions on how to release, and you are also encouraged to design your own. There are so many wonderful moments and years in the life of a family that may depend on conscious awareness and healthy integration now.

Responsibility: No Victims

Healthy integration also requires ultimate responsibility. Gestalt therapy, and most other approaches to mental health, are built on the principle of total responsibility: no victims, just responsible participants. If women, for example, are viewed as victims of obstetrical practices, then we will continue to feel helpless and powerless to change what must be changed and to encourage what must be continued. Physicians and nurses, by their roles in medicine and in the lives of individuals, seek and acquire much power. This power can be used to heal and assist others in locating their own resources for self-healing. It can also be misused to control and to dictate, under the rubric of good practice, rigid standards for medical practice. The misuse can cause much physical violation as well as emotional pain.

As women, we are responsible for whom we bring into our lives and into our birthing rooms. Hopefully, our choices will honor and respect our birthing process and our human dignity. When we give to our physicians omnipotent power, we invite them to control our births and to rescue (as well as persecute) us as the victims. The power of the physician is a paper tiger, a tiger in an iron jail built out of a childhood legacy that has denied our worth and our sense of competence. The more we can free the paper tiger, the more genuine control we have over our choices in childbirth and in our lives.

If we remain victims, angry at our physicians, we risk damage to our own bodies, we further cement the obstetrical unions, and we do to others (victimize them) exactly what we have despised having done to us.

Forgiveness: The Ultimately Practical Act

This view of psychological integration does not excuse the misuse of power, nor does it condone some of the painfully rigid obstetrical practices of today. It does, however, include ultimate forgiveness for all participants in the childbirth drama, so that we can live our lives free from victims (ourselves and others). Although this view may at first glance sound complacent, it is actually effective, active, concerned, and, most of all, psychologically sound, as the chapters ahead will describe.

Susan's Story

The following report was written by a woman intent on positive birthing and on healthy integration. Susan is 30 years old. She lives in a Boston suburb with her husband Mario and their three children. She wrote this report after attending a seminar designed for positive, effective parenting based on healthy integration at childbirth.

> *Interrupting the tomb-like stillness of the room, the leader's [Ken's] voice flowed into my subconscious, forcing reality upon me. I awoke and found myself doubled over on the couch, my head almost into Mario's lap. Ken's hand was on my shoulder, his whispering voice encouraging me to keep breathing. . . . .*
>
> *To the quieting, instrumental sounds of Steve Halpern's "Spectrum Suite," Ken began the guided meditation by counting backwards slowly. "Three . . . two, you are feeling more and more relaxed . . . one . . . allowing yourself the total experience of this birth."*
>
> *I was transported back in time to our tiny apartment, busy hanging the curtains that I had just finished making. As I squatted to fix them, I felt a stream of warm liquid spreading smoothly over my thighs. With the baby's expected due date only a few days away, I knew my water had broken.*
>
> *Feeling both excited and afraid, I went to tell Mario what had happened. He was lying on the living room couch, pale and unshaven. Yesterday afternoon he had been released from the hospital after a serious bout with spinal meningitis.*
>
> *Mario glared at me through sunken eyes as I told him the news, and angrily replied, "Quit fooling around!" Not wanting to upset him further, I turned and left the room. As I reached the door, I heard him dialing the*

phone and listened as he told the doctor what he, himself, had not wanted to hear.

Before leaving for the hospital we phoned my parents. They were excited and asked if I would rather they go with me. I guiltily explained that it was Mario that I wanted beside me.

I resented his being sick. Why now? He was turning greener by the minute, this strong, virile husband of mine. Where was his strength that I had learned to depend on?

We arrived at the hospital in the midst of a great deal of commotion. The hospital was not clear on what to do about Mario. Would the baby contract the meningitis? Mario's doctor was called in as a precaution, and while he gave his okay for Mario to be present, he shot me a disapproving look.

I had arrived at the hospital around 5:00 p.m. with my contractions beginning shortly thereafter. It was now close to 9:00 p.m., and I was finally settled into my room. It was the only prepared childbirth room, decorated with yellow flowered wallpaper and equipped with its own private bathroom and an adjoining sitting room complete with television, magazines, and games. By now my contractions were coming fast and furious, and I wondered, if this was only the beginning, how was I ever going to last the night?

My doctor, who had just arrived at the hospital, poked his head into the room and inquired as to how I was doing. I replied, "Fine," not wanting to sound incompetent, but the contractions were becoming increasingly hard to manage. I had no idea I was in transition. Glancing at my chart while still standing in the doorway, the doctor estimated that, this being my first, I could expect to deliver sometime tomorrow morning. He then went on to tell me that he was leaving to deliver a baby in another hospital a few miles away. My face must have revealed my surprise, for the next thing I knew he was changed out of his street clothes and into hospital garb and was standing at the foot of my bed.

He proceeded to examine me and with a surprised look announced that the baby's head was crowning. Mario knew it was time for him to change into the required garments, and quickly left the room. No sooner had he closed the door when the doctor, trying to hurry the process, reached both his hands up inside of me and proceeded to stretch the birth canal. A muffled scream escaped my lips. He quickly stopped and explained, "It will make the delivery easier for you." Did he really believe I was that naive?

Tears silently rolled down my cheeks. The breathing exercises were totally forgotten as my body filled with hurt and fear.

The doctor called to the nurse for assistance in transporting me to the delivery room. The corridor was cold and dismal as they hurried me along. I looked around for Mario, who was just arriving through the swinging doors. In the cold and brightly lit room I reached out for his hand, and as my gaze slowly arched upwards, I saw that he was as disoriented and afraid as I was. Damn him for not knowing what the doctor had done to me. I could feel pity only for myself.

The nurses rolled me onto my side and held my arms and legs as the anesthesiologist administered a saddleblock. I had requested no anesthetic be given. Why were they discounting me like this? They certainly had no idea of my inner turmoil, for I was playing their game with all I had.

Michael was born as the anesthetic was still taking effect. One nurse glanced at me knowingly as I let my emotions rob me of the moment. But I was not done yet. The doctor, who by now was in a vast hurry, pounced onto my tender abdomen in an effort to push the afterbirth out. A few quick sutures and his job was done.

The nurses bustled around cleaning, weighing, and whatever else it is they do to newborns. Through a weakly mustered smile I asked to hold my baby. They held his tiny body close to me and hurriedly returned to their task. My body ached with the urgency of having him bonded to me. I needed him in my arms!

My body began to tremble. The nurses stopped their busy work to make sympathetic noises and pile me high with warm blankets. I was wheeled out into the dismal, deserted corridor beside the nurses' station. Mario had left to make the phone calls.

It was late, and it seemed like an eternity before my convulsing body quieted down. The young nurse, who was just assigned to me, wheeled me to my room and glanced at my chart. The chart read, "No anesthetic requested." She did not bother to ask if that was truly the case as she sat me on the edge of my bed and later began walking me around. As a result, I woke a few hours later with excruciating head pains. The doctor prescribed codeine, which I refused to take because I was breastfeeding. The headache remained with me for three weeks.

Ken's warm voice began slowly counting, "Three . . . two . . . one . . ."
My eyes gradually opened as I began to feel my presence in the room. The painful memories had caused my body to slump over, my head almost into Mario's lap. Ken's hand was on my shoulder, his soft voice encouraging me to keep breathing. As I looked up into his eyes, he asked me to forgive them all.

I forgave.

After many years of inner guilt toward herself and anger toward her husband and her medical attendants, Susan set herself free. She became free to be open to her marriage, free to seek medical information without anger, and free to experience peace of mind as a childbearing woman. We deserve and need that freedom.

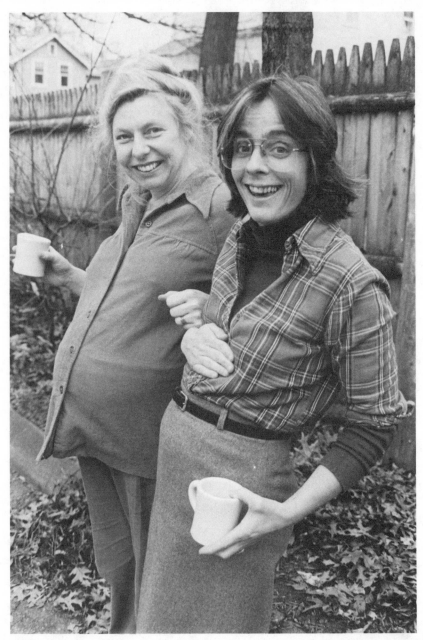

©Peggy McMahon

2

Maternal Well-Being: The Primary Goal

In recent years, the importance of the maternal influence on the family system has been downplayed in an attempt to equalize roles and expectations and to free women of the former deluge of demands that were—and still are—made upon them. However, a mother's influence over the family system is a primary determinant in the functioning and relationship patterns within the family unit. Unfortunately, mothers have been given so little recognition and respect for their work that some of us still tend to feel inadequate and apologetic when we introduce ourselves unless we have some successful career outside our homes in our recent past or some lofty goals for further professional advancement in the future.

It is time that we elevate in our own hearts and minds the position of mother and the job of mothering. It is time that men and women respect and recognize the significance of a mother in the life of each family member.

In *Our Bodies, Ourselves*, the authors have helped to refocus our energies on the importance of the woman as nurturer and to recognize the power, creativity, and beauty in that aspect of us. The authors liberate women from the historical notion that nurturing is a sole or primary aspect of the female make-up and proclaim the totality of women (Boston Women's Health Book Collective 1978b). It is in this context that the importance of maternal well-being will be discussed.

Maternal Well-Being during Childbirth: Long-Term Impact

Maternal well-being—physical, emotional, mental, spiritual—is a must for positive birthing. Without having faith in ourselves and believing that we deserve decent and supported childbearing, we cannot achieve our goals. Maternal well-being as the primary goal in childbearing is a concept built on the belief that childbearing greatly influences the long-term psychological condition of the family system. Helene Deutsch recognized this relationship of events back in the 1940s in her work *The Psychology of Women* (1945). She wrote, "The main problems of motherhood make their appearance at the beginning of the reproductive function and, as we have seen, continue, with the birth of the child, in the mother's relation to him."

Judith Duncan (1982) indicated that follow-up interviews of postpartum women tended to reflect a stronger sense of guilt and inadequacy about mothering in those women who tended to express guilt or failure feelings about their childbirths. Lewis Mehl and Gayle Peterson (1979) studied the emotional effects of childbearing on women. They confirmed a relationship between a woman's ability to actively participate in her childbirth experience (with adequate preparation and support) and her gaining in personal self-confidence and overall mental health as a result of her birthing experience. Most readers would agree that improved self-confidence and overall mental health could only serve to improve maternal-child relationships.

Woman—Value Thyself!

Some may view the emphasized need for maternal well-being as selfish. They may fear that children will suffer as a result or feel that too much is being made of a normal, everyday event. To the first of these, it is agreed. It *is* selfish, and it is time women (especially mothers) *became* selfish. Many American women were brought up in families where mealtimes meant that the entire family ate and the women cleaned up afterwards; where girls baby-sat for younger siblings, while boys of equal age and ability played ball; or where the social, educational, and/or athletic needs of male children were considered of greater value than those of female children. Mother's Day was the day on which men treated women the same way women treated men all year—cooking and serving a special meal, etc.

To demonstrate the results of such practices, women, mostly mothers, are often asked in our seminars how many of them urinate within two minutes of the time they first receive a physical impulse to do so—and almost no one responds. However, when asked how many of them wait until they feel desperate to go, an overwhelming majority lift their hands. (This is, perhaps, a contributing factor in the high rate of bladder infections in women!) How can a culture of women who have been socialized to wait until we are desperate to *urinate,* speak up for our needs during *childbearing?* Only through an absolute overhaul of our present thinking patterns.

Sex Role Scripting

Claude Steiner and Hogie Wycoff, authors of *Scripts People Live* (1974), have described several of the basic life scripts common to the American woman. "Script," a term coined by Eric Berne (1972), defines life patterns as ongoing dramas with plots, characters, and settings that become enacted in daily life. Wycoff believes that women are "trained to accept the mystification that they are imcomplete, inadequate, and dependent," as the following scripts indicate (Steiner 1974):

> *Mother Hubbard* is the woman who spends her life nurturing others and sees herself as the least important family member and chronically feels unappreciated. She is run by inner voices that tell her to "be a good mother," "be nice" and "sacrifice for others."
>
> *The Woman behind the Man* is the woman who puts her life energy into supporting her male partner in a way that discounts her own talent and ability. She is probably most typically found in the Politician or Doctor's wife and is run by inner voices telling her to be helpful and not take credit.
>
> *Poor Little Me* is the woman who grows up in a family where women are viewed as helpless and inadequate. With a body that tends to be weak and off-balance, her inner voices tell her to discount her ability to think for herself.
>
> *Tough Lady* is an independent woman taught by her family not to trust or count on others. She is afraid to ask for or receive help and spends her life proving she can survive alone. This script is the flip side of the helpless, dependent life patterns but is not based on true independence or self-confidence.

These scripts are decided upon in early childhood and are often based on imcomplete, misleading, or inaccurate information. The starring roles and prototype dramas are often derived from fairy-tale plots such as Cinderella, Sleeping Beauty, Snow White, Little Red Riding Hood, and Goldilocks. All too often, we are faced with a plot that involves the main character's self-sacrificing nature, an evil witch or stepmother, and a male rescuer who saves all.

Today's Woman

The modern-day reenactment of these fairy tales is discussed in Colette Dowling's bestseller, *The Cinderella Complex* (1981), in which the author discusses how women fail to respect their own intuitive, intellectual and mental decision-making powers, how we back down from challenge and seek to be saved. In childbearing practices, one can perhaps better understand how midwives became synonymous with witches, such as the one who offered a poison apple to Snow White. The historical practice of punishing women as witches for their healing powers and these modern-day fairy tales have led, as Suzanne Arms (1975) writes, to a deception in childbearing that devalues the skill of the midwife and leaves consumers in fear of some association with witchcraft. It may also help to explain why so many "prepared" women who attended childbirth education courses, read extensively, and faithfully practiced body and breathing exercises still find themselves seeking the physician (the handsome or not-so-handsome prince) in times of perceived or real crisis in delivery, rather than their own inner resources and intuitive drives toward self-healing (which may or may not include taking medical interventions).

Others fear that children would in some way suffer if maternal well-being were to become the primary goal in the childbearing process. Samuels and Bennett (1974) describe the concept of well-being as "the body's natural abilities for self-regulation and inborn healing." They repeatedly suggest that "health" is maintained when one is freed from external pressures and internal upsets, which block the natural tendency toward health and aliveness. The goal of individual well-being, as they view it, is essential to the avoidance of disease and the maintaining of health. This description of well-being is based on the idea that well-being is instinctive and that the being tends toward health unless interrupted. In the first chapter, improved maternal and infant health through proper nutrition and prenatal diet were discussed, emphasizing the fact that it is much easier for the psychologically healthy, emotionally aware woman to believe in the importance of caring for her body and to have the psychic energy necessary to produce healthy daily eating habits. Improved mental well-being allows for a natural flow of intuition and love as demonstrated in the drive for maternal-infant protection. Women are instinctively and intuitively directed toward the health and well-being of their children. A look at the animal kingdom demonstrates that personal self-preservation (a primary drive in all animals, including humans) yields only when there is a threat to the life of the offspring or when some abnormality (disturbance in well-being) blocks natural drives. The mother deer, for instance, runs from its predators unless a fawn is endangered. In those instances, she fights to the point of sacrificing herself in order to save her young. The human mother develops a protective response during pregnancy that causes her to cover her stomach and protect the fetus when danger is perceived. Further, it is this instinctive and loving protective force that allows women to so easily surrender to the dangers and, sometimes, disappointments of Cesarean deliveries in an attempt to save their children's lives. It is ironic that sectioned mothers should ever be viewed as weak or inadequate after the heroics and self-sacrifice of a Cesarean delivery. More on this in later chapters. The point is that maternal well-being supports life—life of mother and life of child.

Bonding

There also seems to be a strong urge for closeness and intimacy between parents and children at the time of birth. This drive is again demonstrated in the animal kingdom. Harlow and Harlow in their famous work with Rhesus monkeys (1966) noted a strong preference in infant monkeys for mothers and mother-like objects, with less apparent behavior conflicts in monkeys who bonded with their specie mother. Klaus and Kennell (1982) observed the importance of maternal-infant bonding and early closeness and noted behavior advantages for bonded infants up to one year after birth. It is this same drive toward intimacy that has led consumers to seek rooming-in and more family-centered birthing practices, and again, it is proposed that maternal well-being is the source of this drive.

Bonding for Love, not Guilt

It should be noted here that these studies on bonding are presented only to emphasize the natural desire for maternal-infant closeness and the greater tendency toward bonding in a psychologically and physically healthy mother. It is necessary to recognize that, yes, bonding is important. However, far too many parents have used these studies to blame themselves for some permanent damage or disservice done to their children by a lack of physical bonding within a so-called critical hour after birth. One does not produce a psychological basket-case because of maternal-infant separation:

> The pressure to do everything "right," and the concept of a brief critical period at birth for bonding, have placed extra burdens on young mothers and fathers. On top of this, current over-emphasis on immediate reinforcement, or offering the right response at the right time, diminishes the composure and confidence of new parents [Brazelton 1981].

Bonding studies have been primarily done with animals and institutionalized children with rather severe deprivation compared to the normal child. As Brazelton reminds us, these studies often do not account for human intellectual and creative capacities for change.

In any case, the natural tendency toward closeness between parents and children seems evident throughout the animal kingdom. Natural states are magnetic forces when well-being is at work (Bennett & Samuels 1974).

Maternal well-being in this context can only lead to improved infant well-being.

Conscious Childbirth

Finally, there are those who would say that childbearing is a normal, everyday event and that this whole book is too much psychological ado about nothing. This attitude of unconsciousness has only impeded the much-needed changes in childbirth preparation and further supported the continuation of emotionally upsetting obstetrical practices that fail to understand the psychological impact of childbirth.

Helene Deutsch (1945) stressed the psychological stresses and changes of childbearing women. "Motherhood as an individual experience is the expression not only of a biologic process, but also of psychologic unity that epitomizes numerous individual experiences, memories, wishes and fears that have preceded the real experience by many years." Deutsch also described the emotional needs of women during this process and recognized the profound need for increased mothering on the part of women during this time.

Normal Stress

Sheila Kitzinger, in her work *The Experience of Childbirth* (1981), wrote a manual of physical and emotional preparation for the expectant mother, saying, "A woman is not just a machine through which a baby is brought to birth by the doctor or midwife . . . .

. . . efficiency is important but the body is a part of the person for whom the birth of the baby is of major emotional significance."

Dr. Grete Bibring (1961), psychoanalyst and researcher on motherhood, speaks of childbearing as a maturational event much like adolescence. She reminds us of the irreversible aspect of motherhood, which does not allow anyone to be relieved of her new role. Who among us passed gracefully through adolescence without great psychological changes? The literature abounds with recognition of the depth of conscious and unconscious processing that women must do in order to successfully integrate the events of birth. The chapters ahead will further explore the depth of emotional impact on the female psyche that childbirth brings from the ordinary, normal vaginal delivery to the more complicated premature deliveries and Cesarean sections, as well as fetal and infant losses. For now, it is important to say that this discussion of psychological impact does not imply any abnormal or pathological condition but rather a very normal condition of psychological awareness experienced by very healthy, conscious women. Unfortunately, too many women define themselves as crazy or abnormal for their consciousness.

Opportunity for Growth

Normal childbearing is a combination of agony and ecstasy. It offers women great opportunity for personal growth and transformation. Equally, it presents opportunities for guilt, inner suffering, and hurt. Yes, childbirth is normal and healthy. It is also profoundly emotional, deeply spiritual, and highly stressful. Remaining conscious and aware of one's feelings during this time insures genuine joy and celebration of childbirth and allows for release of all painful feelings in a responsible way, regardless of the external events.

Anne's Story

Failure to remain conscious and aware may cause much hurt and conflict for many years to follow. Anne's post-birth experience amplifies this point.

Anne, age 27, had planned a hospital birth at a suburban hospital in Rhode Island. This was her first pregnancy and one that she and her husband had planned for almost two years. She felt that she was not psychologically prepared to assume the risks of a home birth. (She made an interesting point about this issue in that she believed that if her baby was injured or died in a hospital setting she could always blame the doctor. However, if the same event happened at home, she would blame herself. How common that we would need a target of blame in order to insure psychological balance, although the choice of birthplace is still to be respected.)

Anne's labor went very well. She, her husband, and labor attendant entered the hospital exactly as she planned, at 7 centimeters. Her physician met her, examined her, and gave her strong, positive reports that she felt provided much-needed encouragement. Four hours later her child was born, a daughter, Janie. She received no drugs, no preps, and no episiotomy, and she tore only slightly. She noticed that she was very tired from the birth and felt a strong urge to rest with her baby daughter at her side.

However, Anne had seen several movies in childbirth education of women laughing, energized by birth, and she believed that she should look exactly the same way. Anne stated that she looked like a washed-out dish rag. She wanted her husband to stay and massage her body but did not want to interfere with his "fun" of calling the relatives, etc. Her husband left, Anne fell asleep, and secretly internalized her tiredness as not loving her baby enough to stay awake.

Four months after Janie's birth, Anne came for counseling. She was not sure why but knew she really needed it. After five sessions, it was suggested that whatever she was paying herself back for had been taken care of and that she had no further debt to pay. She burst into tears and said that she was embarrassed to tell anyone that she fell asleep after the birth and did not look at all like the women in the movies, and that she was still angry that her husband had left to make phone calls. She had not wanted to resume her former marital sex life, which she said had been quite good, and she did not attend her follow-up childbirth class with her baby because she thought someone would see that she did not love Janie enough. Anne was a normal, healthy woman. She was tired after birth and needed to be massaged (a postpartum ritual common in some sections of India) and to sleep (a natural state of recuperation).

Once Anne was able to release her fears and hurts, she resumed her sex life and began to speak about Janie's birth with a sense of self-affirmation and genuine celebration. She shared her story with several women friends and said she was amazed to discover that others had similar fears and self-criticisms, and that her well-kept secrets were common feelings to many women who, like herself, felt they could not share the agonies of childbearing and so were forced to fake the ecstasies—thereby missing out on the growth and expansion inherent in accepting all aspects. Anne is in the company of many women who fear that they are abnormal, inadequate, or crazy because they are conscious, healthy, and alive. Let us support this psychological health and aliveness. Let us make maternal well-being our priority right now.

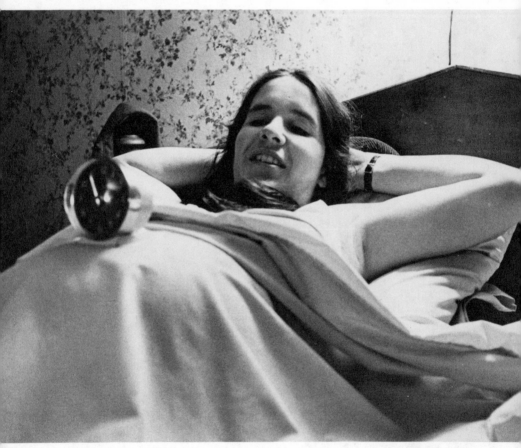

3

Five Key Attitudes
for Positive Birthing

Helene Deutsch (1945) wrote, "The psychosomatic interdependence of the psychologic and physiologic processes is nowhere so clearly demonstrated as in the female reproduction activity." She knew well the profound relationship of mind and body and the manifestation of this relationship in childbearing.

Many theories of psychotherapy and healing are built on the principle that the mind influences the body. Alexander Lowen (1975) in his work on bioenergetics described how one's body is an expression of one's state of mind. A rigid, conflicted mental state that lacks trust expresses itself in a tight, rigid physical structure, that may emanate the message, "Leave me alone." Conversely, a peaceful, happier mental state is reflected in a more relaxed physical body structure.

Mind Influences Body

Sondra Ray, in her book *Loving Relationships* (1980), and Jim Morningstar, in *Spiritual Psychology* (1980), describe how thought carries energy, which is read in the body and in the physical world. They suggest, for example, that if one carries the thought, "Money is the root of all evil," financial problems may result in order to avoid the evil. Or, if one has the thought, "Men hurt me," this may unconsciously attract certain obstetrical practices. Simply stated, in their system, we get what we think.

25

Morningstar emphasizes the power of thought over body function. To illustrate this point, he describes how the Trobriand Islanders use thought as a form of birth control. The islanders believe that one can only become pregnant within the context of marriage. Although there is much premarital intercourse, pregnancy occurs only within marriage. I do not recommend thought as a form of birth control for Western-reared couples; however, the influence over the reproductive function in Trobriand Islanders certainly speaks to the point (Morningstar 1980).

John Diamond, M.D., in his work in biokinesiology (1980), a study of the body as an electric system, demonstrates through muscle tensing and relaxing the influence of thoughts over the condition of the body. If a subject is asked to tighten the muscles of an outstretched arm and think of a happy time, the arm remains strong and is able to resist the outside pressure of someone pushing down on the flexed muscle. However, if that same subject is asked to think of a time when he or she felt hurt or upset, the flexed arm loses force and succumbs to outside pressure. Should the subject persist in negative thinking, all muscle tone will virtually disappear, clearly demonstrating the power of negative thinking over the body's natural strength and aliveness.

Mind Power and Disease

In recent years, the theories of body-mind integration have been applied to the treatment of disease and injury. The Simontons, in their work *Getting Well Again* (1978), describe how cancer patients can actively participate in the treatment of their illness and achieve some very positive outcomes in prolonged life expectancies, rapid remissions, and, in some cases, total cures. Norman Cousins, in *The Anatomy of an Illness as Told by the Patient* (1979), told of his own personal self-cure through positive attitudes and alternatives to traditional treatment. Afflicted with a progressive disease of the connective tissue, Cousins signed himself out of a hospital and into a hotel. Remaining under a physician's care, he ate healthily, took vitamins to regain his physical strength, and used laughter and positive thinking to reduce pain and repair damaged tissue.

Mind in Childbirth

Although the earliest pioneers in prepared childbirth, such as Lamaze and Dick-Read, based their works on mind-body connections, it is only in more recent years that the actual mental influence over birthing outcomes has been researched and acknowledged. Gayle Peterson and Lewis Mehl describe in detail the use of mind-body integration during childbearing. In her book *Birthing Normally* (1981) Peterson suggests the use of psychological interventions such as support rather than the usual medical interferences that may alleviate one problem but give rise to another (e.g., Pitocin, which induces or increases labor but often leads to pain medications because of the interference with normal build-up of tolerance to labor pain). Peterson writes that "the body-mind integration is the most effective force in affecting change."

Most writers on the subject of childbearing would agree that childbearing is a time of great change, physically and emotionally. Because it is such a transitional period, it is an opportune time for women to rethink their former beliefs, values, and attitudes and to replace any historical mental systems that are not devoted to total well-being with new mental attitudes that are.

Mind and Stress

As childbearing produces stress, it is an optimum time for learning. In *Magical Child* (1977), Joseph Chilton Pearce describes how normal stress is not only conducive to learning but also a requirement. Pearce says, "The unknown—unpredictable—imposes sensory data that do not fit the brain's established editorial policies well enough to be handled automatically by various subordinates." He goes on to describe how the entire system goes on alert and becomes more available to receive new data. This tendency toward change and perhaps improvement is demonstrated in the physical and psychical overhaul common to pregnant couples. For example, it is not uncommon for the pregnant woman to read volumes on diet and health care, labor and delivery, infant and postpartum care. Most women will alter their diet (to the degree of integrated maternal well-being) and attempt to eat healthily. This is a time when couples give up smoking and alcohol and cut down on coffee, sugar, and red meat. Women often engage in a new exercise, such as walking or swimming. Couples tend to do a self-imposed critique of their present marriage relationship and attempt to alleviate areas of stress and conflict. It seems, then, an ideal time to introduce attitudes conducive to both positive birthing and positive living. The following discussion focuses on five attitudes essential for positive childbearing.

Five Essential Attitudes

Self-Love

In Western culture, we are raised on a legacy of disapproval and approval that creates inner voices of criticism and perfectionistic demands. Muriel James calls this process "conditional love," where a child is loved for her ability to conform or perform rather than for her essence as a human being (James & Jongeward 1973). We are trained not to "brag" or say good things about ourselves for fear of becoming selfish, swell-headed, or egocentric.

Marshall Summer says, "Egotism is trying to prove that you are okay after you've fallen into hating yourself" (Ray 1980). Even when we do have a sense of self-love, it is usually based on an illusion of feeling good rather than real inner peace. We attempt to gain it by doing well enough, or by accomplishing enough. This system is probably best exemplified in our relationships with our own bodies. In one of my classes, a woman shared with us the significant fact that, a year earlier, she had given up getting on a scale. It was her liberation day: previously, she used to get on a scale every day. If she weighed 120 pounds, she decided that she was a completely okay, lovable person. If she weighed 125 pounds, she decided she was a disgusting, out-of-control person who was completely worthless. Between 121 and 124, she could go either way. On the days that she weighed 120 pounds, she was temporarily fine—until she ate an extra piece of bread. Her total sense of well-being crashed at 125 pounds, and, like most women (and men), scales were not the only place she was mentally grading herself on her performance.

Far too many Western women find themselves trying to prove something about themselves in childbirth rather than trying to love themselves. This inner demand for performance and perfection leads women to focus their energies on doing well at breathing during labor rather than on the genuine physical needs and messages offered by their own bodies. Far too many women mentally grade themselves for perfect weight gain rather than love themselves with proper nutrition. We grade ourselves on our ability to have carefree pregnancies rather than allow a full range of inner emotions, and we grade ourselves on how we deliver our children rather than celebrate ourselves for our courage to birth. The real question is not, "Have you done your breathing exercises?" but rather, "Can you love yourself no matter how you birth, where you birth, or what the outcome?"

In the previous chapter, female programing in caring for others, ignoring ourselves, and discounting our ability to think for ourselves was discussed. Reactions to these scripts have caused us to become super-independent, super-self-sufficient, and completely able to do everything. Both of these positions—the adapted, helpless, powerless child and the over-independent superwoman—lead us away from ourselves. They are positions still founded on fear of disapproval and ultimate obligation.

It is true that self-love is a large goal, but when applied to daily living it becomes, perhaps, a series of smaller goals. Self-love leads to maternal well-being, as the following story may help to explain.

Betty, a seminar participant, shared that she had worked herself into physical exhaustion before the birth of her first child by going to parties

over the Christmas holidays and having guests whom she did not really want
to entertain. Betty was almost 30 and a practicing attorney who lived just
outside of Worcester, Massachusetts. By the time she went into labor, she
was exhausted and had a very difficult time laboring and recovering from
her birth. Now she was pregnant for the second time and in her eighth
month. Her sister and her sister's children were due to stay at Betty's for
a week's vacation. Although Betty wanted to tell her sister not to come, she
felt obligated and afraid of her sister's anger. During the seminar she decided
that her physical and mental rest were more important than avoiding her
sister's anger, and Betty decided to call and cancel.

Eight weeks later Betty sent a letter describing her birth. She felt so
pleased with herself for saying No to her sister that she continued to take
care of herself, guided by her bodily needs, right up through her birth. She
wrote, "Once I told my sister I needed to rest, I could also tell my friends
and other family members. In fact, I even told my doctor no episiotomy
when he offered one. I told him, 'I'm stretchable—a one-size-fits-all!'
Thanks. . . . P.S. I didn't tear."

Intention to Succeed

Intention to succeed means that we remind ourselves regularly that we
are whole, competent human beings. For a long time, Western women have
been programmed in noncompetence. Dorothy Jongeward, in *Women as
Winners*, describes the stroking patterns common to women, that is, the
behaviors for which women are most likely to receive acknowledgement
(Jongeward & Scott 1976). The patterns demonstrate a strong tendency in
women to discount their own ability to think and decide for themselves and,
instead, to adapt to whatever expectations are presented by the primary
figures in the environment. The result of this training is evident in the top-
heavy *male* executive population in both business and in government.

It is still acceptable for a woman not to be able to balance a checkbook,
change a tire, or fill out an income tax form. When a man is unable to do
these tasks, he is more likely to be defined, or to define himself, as weak,
inadequate, and incompetent. There are different views about women as
athletes that tend to undermine female athletic interest and ability by de-
fining it as whimsical play or liberated flexing. Males engaged in the same
sports, such as basketball, baseball, or hockey, are viewed as serious players.

Intention to succeed means believing in oneself wholeheartedly. Again,
this does not mean that any goal in childbirth is more important than maternal well-being and birthing, or that any event or outcome should be
viewed as failure. It does, however, suggest that we as women define ourselves as capable. It is interesting to notice that Sandra O'Connor's appointment to the Supreme Court was met with headlines that announced "A

Woman on the Bench!" as though O'Connor had overcome her basic defect as a woman in order to be appointed. Her abilities and competence were secondary. We would not say, "Samuel O'Connor has been appointed, and he's a man!" What is expected of men is still unexpected of women.

Many childbirth educators recommend that women bring their husbands to their obstetrical appointments in order to get the information they are seeking. This concept is built on the notion that a physician will treat a man with a kind of dignity and respect that he will not give to a woman. If you as a woman are prepared to speak on behalf of yourself and to ask the questions you need to ask, then you deserve the same respect, dignity, and answers your husband or male partner would get. If you are not getting your own answers, you have the wrong physician. You should not need a male partner to validate your credibility and should only seek physicians who treat you decently and with dignity in all matters. Otherwise, you are bringing to your child's birth an energy that does not believe in you, that anticipates failure and defines you as incapable right from the start. Suzanne Arms, in *Immaculate Deception* (1975), writes, "That many women feel they have failed in one way or another in their births is not due to the method they practice but to the expectation of failure built into every hospital staff." She is referring here to education practices and medical testimonies about women "attempting" or "trying" natural childbirth, rather than assumptions of competence and ability. Gayle Peterson, in *Birthing Normally* (1981), says, "In the case of childbirth, the client gives away her responsibility to the practitioner, along with the power to correct the situation." She reminds professionals that birth is stress and that interventions should only come in distress, otherwise they undermine a woman's confidence in herself.

Robert Mendelsohn, M.D. (1981), describes birthing rooms and reminds women that these wallpapered hospital rooms are still expressions of medical interference and lack of faith in women's ability to give birth. Hidden in the tidy dresser drawers are the obstetrician's tools for robbing women of their ability to birth—perhaps in a more frightening way than in the delivery room, where the reminders of unnecessary intervention are more obvious. Intention to succeed through faith in ourselves can only come from within. The conditioning for failure is rampant, although unconscious, in obstetrics, and requires an attitude of conscious awareness.

Conscious Awareness

Recently, at a week-long workshop, my 4½-year-old son walked up to a black woman participant and asked her why her skin was so brown. He asked her if she had any white spots anywhere and why her teeth were white. Although my son had met blacks before, he was in a live-in workshop setting that supported consciousness and apparently felt safe enough to ask.

Although I like to think of myself as enlightened, I felt embarrassed and awkward in the face of his questions.

Two days later he asked a male participant with a severe stuttering problem why he could not talk. The man responded kindly and explained his stuttering problem. Throughout the week my son expressed his impatience and anger at Steve for stuttering, but seemed to clear it up and go on each time to play with Steve without upset. No adult participants shared their anger, upset, or impatience in the same way. Again, I wanted to view myself as enlightened, and again, I was humiliated by my son's openness, although pleased as well.

My son's conscious expression of curiosity and anger serve to remind us of how secretive and unconscious we really are. We are still a culture that cries, burps, and passes gas in the bathroom so no one will see us, and that expresses anger only when we are desperately resentful and bitter. Childbirth is another area of unconsciousness. Burdened by picture-perfect birth scenes, couples are often unable to share the true depth of joy or the depth of hurt, disappointment, anger, or grief.

Although we like to think of ourselves as open-minded, we tend to revert to the familiar. We often eat the same food for breakfast, wear the same hairstyle, and continue to use the same physician, whether our needs are being met or not. Once we develop a habit pattern, we often find change difficult and conscious awareness impossible, as evidenced by the millions of cigarette smokers who cannot consciously connect to the fact that they are killing themselves.

We tend to be more interested in matching our mental pictures than in evaluating relationships and situations. Conscious awareness allows us to evaluate present needs and desires and to adequately prepare for the realities of labor, including pain, fear, and discomfort as well as challenge, joy, and release. It allows us to view each birth experience as a unique event and to discover the experience of each moment in childbirth. Ina May Gaskin (1977) reminds us to "stay conscious because it takes intelligence to give birth."

We are critical of physicians who put our bodies to sleep with drugs; let us not put our feelings to sleep with attitudes of unconscious awareness. Lyn Delliquadri and Kati Breckenridge comment (1979), "Conscious knowing puts you in control of your behavior. For instance, if you are aware of a hole in the ground, you can choose whether you want to step in it or not. If you are not aware of it, your fate is no longer your decision and you may end up with a sprained ankle."

Responsibility

In Chapter Two, female scripts that support women as victims were discussed. The fairy-tale prototypes in Cinderella, Sleeping Beauty, and

Snow White support the "Poor Little Me" position that renders women victims of their surroundings and, most of all, of themselves. Steve Karpman defined life dramas in a triangular motion based on three predominant roles: the Rescuer (commonly portrayed as the good guy or gal in the white hat), who must save the underdog; the Persecutor (commonly portrayed as the bad guy or gal in the black hat), who unjustly injures or violates the underdog; and the Victim, who must give up all sense of personal power and become helplessly out of control (Steiner 1974).

As long as women resort to damsel-in-distress routines during childbirth, the Persecutors and Rescuers will continue to interfere. It becomes difficult to distinguish the Rescuers from the Persecutors in that the former assume lack of ability in the Victim in the same way that the Persecutor assumes the right to violate the victim.

Helen Marieskind, in a 1979 report to the U.S. Department of Health, Education and Welfare, described the twelve reasons for the high rate of Cesarean section in the United States today. The first reason is fear of malpractice suits. Physicians are, frankly, covering themselves for all possible contingencies, a natural outcome of the present obstetrical dramas. The Karpman dramas have movement and the roles are flexible, so that as long as physicians want to be the Rescuers and women the damsels-in-distress, childbirth will be an arena for malpractice as the Victim becomes the Persecutor and the Rescuer the Victim—all feeling wronged and violated. The biggest Victim is always the winner. So this is a game in which one loses much in order to win.

Dramas need scapegoats. Scapegoats mean blame and blame means lack of responsibility. There may be times when lawsuits would be legitimate outcomes of genuine malpractice that requires correction. There may be other times, however, when our own feelings of failure or guilt cause us to assign blame, pass judgment, and seek revenge.

Sondra Ray, in *Loving Relationships Training* (1980), says that if you are looking for advice you are probably looking for someone to blame if things do not go well—which already assumes that things will not go well. Gayle Peterson (1981) writes that the more a woman excuses her behavior as the result of being a victim, the more practiced she becomes at viewing herself as not responsible for her life events. Labor becomes an event, one in which she can easily fall into the trap of passivity in the victim role. Nancy Cohen and Lois Estner, in *Silent Knife* (1983), remind us "Birth is for women, not girls," and point out that childbearing is an opportunity to grow ourselves up fast and assume the challenges of the experience. It is an opportunity to give up our scapegoats and damsel-in-distress routines and respond to ourselves with competence, strength, assurance—genuine "response-ability."

Women as Wonderful

Some Western families still place a greater value on male children than on female children. A boy will "carry on the family name," whereas a girl will "cost her father a wedding." In earlier chapters, I discussed some of the scripting of females and the painful results of these in childbearing. "Women as wonderful" reflects an attitude not only of equality but of deep personal value associated with one's femaleness. This sense of value is reflected in body images that are supportive of childbearing. Sondra Ray (1980) says, "If you don't love your body, then you don't love yourself." If there is any left-over programing that supports a negative female value system, the body will be a primary reflection of this negative system.

Gayle Peterson (1981) cites, as an example, a woman who suffered ineffective labor and uterine inertia as a result of ambivalent feelings toward her own body. Her inner lack of faith in her physical functioning might have led to medical intervention, had she not been able to change her attitude and reinterpret her physical body as a lovable and effective organism.

In the next chapter, negative female images in terms of historical traditions and familial beliefs in childbearing will be discussed. These images can reflect conflict and stress in the mind and body that can be manifested in pregnancy, labor, and/or delivery.

Here, because birth is such a powerful physical experience, it is important to celebrate ourselves as women—with the women's bodies that produce the miracle of birth. Adrienne Rich, in her book *Of Woman Born* (1976), sums up as follows:

> Childbirth is (or may be) one aspect of the entire process of a woman's life, beginning with her expulsion from her mother's body, her own sexual suckling or being held by a woman, through her earliest sensations of clitoral eroticism and of the vulva as a source of pleasure, her growing sense of her own body and its strengths, her masturbation, her menses, her physical relationship to nature and to other human beings, her first and subsequent orgasmic experiences with another's body, her conception, pregnancy, to the moment of first holding her child.

Since childbearing clearly magnifies our relationship with our physical body, it offers us the opportunity to love each and every part. Any rejection we send psychologically to our own body carries a negative energy. Conversely, every positive, loving thought we send to the physical body carries a positive, healing energy.

Pregnancy is an opportunity to send our best thoughts to all parts of our bodies. It's a good time to *throw away* our scales, eat nutritiously, and let go of hurting and judging ourselves for our shapes!!!

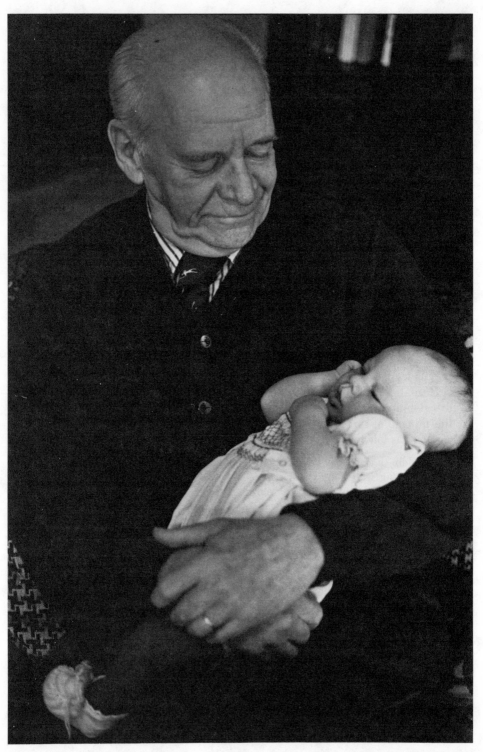

4

Personal History: The Past and Its Influences on Childbearing

Childbearing is an emotionally charged, highly activating event that demands adjustment to change on all levels—physical, mental, emotional, and spiritual. The events and adjustments of childbearing are influenced not only by our present attitudes but also by our historical concepts and thoughts that are stored in each individual human mind and are a combination of each person's unique internalization of pregnancy and of childbirth.

The human mind has a remarkable capacity for storage of data, although only a very limited portion is available to the conscious mind at any given time. The information contained is sometimes inaccurate and based on early childhood decisions that were arrived at through limited experience and inaccurate perception, as discussed in Chapter One. Eric Berne (1972) described this accumulated information as the basis for one's decisions about oneself, others, and the world. He described the human personality in three specific aspects, called "ego states." In Berne's framework, we live in a child ego state for many years before we develop an accurate fact gatherer (an "adult ego state") and a self-protecting energy (a "parent"). Within this child ego state are many emotionally charged events that may be the basis for global decisions. For example, in the life of a child one pregnant woman having a difficult time may become the essence of all pregnancies, leading the child to assume that pregnancy is a difficult and painful time for all women everywhere.

The Influence of Belief Systems

Much has been written about the influence of our thoughts and beliefs over our physical bodies and relationships in the world. Some of this material was discussed in the previous chapter in order to emphasize the importance of positive attitudes in creating positive emotional outcomes. Gayle Peterson and Lewis Mehl have based their psychophysiological approach to childbirth on the principle, "Women birth as they live"; therefore, childbearing is an expression of a woman's beliefs about life (Peterson 1981). Mehl, in his paper "The Importance of Belief in the Childbearing Process" (1979), noted that "affectively charged beliefs create the person's reality." This is particularly true in pregnancy and childbirth, since this whole transitional time is so activating. Nancy Cohen and Lois Estner, in *Silent Knife* (1983), describe pregnancy as a highly charged emotional time. "Pregnancy encompasses a myriad of feelings: fear, joy, excitement, exhaustion, strength. . . . Pregnancy is a catalyst not just for issues about babies, but also about love, caring, finance, security, sexuality."

In essence, childbearing sets off many emotionally charged memories in our mental computer banks, memories that might otherwise remain unconscious and out of awareness. We do not experience pregnancy or childbirth in a vacuum, disconnected from other life events. Life and birth reflect many aspects and conditions of the past. It is important to note here that the mind not only stores memories of events, but also does so in a somewhat organized manner. As children, we do not have a conceptual framework for gathering data. In Eric Berne's terms, we have not yet developed an adult ego state—an objective, neutral, fact gatherer. We therefore must rely on emotional impact as a means of sorting data (Berne 1972). A common early life experience, for example, might be one of loss or separation from parents. This might even have occurred shortly after birth, given the childbearing practices of the 1930s to 1960s, where mother and child were often routinely cared for in separate rooms by strangers. This loss, then, becomes the foundation of future losses that might occur, such as losing a pet, moving to a new town and leaving friends, changing teachers, separation or divorce of parents. These losses will vary from person to person because each of us has such a unique set of life experiences. According to Berne, these experiences will be stored in the mental computer in a set of feelings labeled "losses." This set of feelings, then, is a lifetime of similar events stacked and filed according to emotional impact. The events may be stored as simple memory or may have unreleased emotional charge still attached. A person with a loss stack, as described, might lose a job and become very sad and depressed as an adult in a way that might seem inappropriate. He or she might engage in what seems to be a prolonged grieving process that prevents any attempt at securing a new job. This grieving process is probably an expression of mental health, in that much previously withheld sorrow now has an opportunity for release. When the psychological experience is respected and supported, there is great opportunity for a mental housecleaning of loss stacks and emotional release of historical feelings.

Birth: A Transitional Life Process

In addition to categorizing events according to emotion, we also tend to have a filing system for major life events (e.g., death, birth, marriage, retirement). These transitional events often set off many emotions because holistic change is required, and the psyche must make appropriate adjustments.

Pregnancy and childbirth activate historical stacks. Some of these stacks might be highly supportive to positive birthing, containing good feelings and beliefs about childbearing as a natural, healthy event. Others may contain more painful, hurtful feelings or frightening ideas about childbearing. As in the example of loss stacks, there is often great opportunity for release of emotions and changing of ideas. The tendency toward release is a tendency toward health and well-being, not a signal of mental disturbance or pathology.

In the past five years of childbirth counseling, hundreds of women have expressed to us fears of being crazy, out of control, or mentally incompetent, because of the emotional upheaval and wealth of memory available during the childbearing process. Many women are written off by their family and friends as "just pregnant" and irrational, with very little genuine understanding of the opportunity to release old hurts and find greater mental peace. In the light of health, this psychological process is just another natural inclination to adequately prepare for birthing and parenting. It is a process that deserves our highest support—not patronization and ridicule.

In our counseling experiences over the past several years, we have discovered three areas of life experiences commonly reactivated in the life of childbearing couples, particularly women. These three areas include one's personal birth, family traditions about childbearing, and adolescent sexuality and body image.

Personal Birth: The Psychological Impact on Childbearing

Pre-Leboyer births were not the conscious, welcoming experiences that we prepare and pray for today. Infants were thrust into brightly lit, noisy rooms where birth was (and still is) a hospital procedure rather than a miracle of life. Mothers were routinely medicated, leaving most of us at the mercy of drugs. Infants were often greeted with forceps rather than loving arms. While we were cold, wet, and naked our cords were cut, usually too early, and we were slapped on the backside as a reminder to breathe. Prior to Klaus's extensive studies on bonding (Kennell & Klaus 1976, 1982), we were probably separated from our mothers while we were further violated with silver nitrate—now found to be a potential cause of cataracts and given because of the assumed potential for veneral disease in all women. As Leboyer (1974) has noted, there was no recognition of the physical sensitivities or the emotional capacity of the infant.

Throughout this time, fathers waited—sometimes several floors away—feeling helpless and inadequate as their women partners labored and birthed with strangers.

These conditions might not have been traumatic for each person but were (and still are in some cases) an extremely nonconscious approach to birthing, an approach that permeated the treatment of the mother and the role of the father. This nonconsciousness has caused physical and emotional separation at a time when togetherness of parents and infants, husbands and wives is much needed.

The Psychoanalytic Explanation

As far back as Sigmund Freud, psychotherapists have understood that birth has a psychological impact on the life of the individual. Freud (1932) said that birth caused an "anxiety condition" that resulted in unresolved dependence. Otto Rank (1929) described birth as a rude interruption to uterine life and believed that the individual could spend his/her whole life trying to recover from it. He ascribed great significance to this early trauma, and believed that through our mental reconstructions we are directly acquainted with the fear of being born—particularly women approaching delivery.

The Rebirther's View

In more recent times, the work of Leonard Orr in rebirthing (the use of a yoga-like breathing process for the purpose of healing birth trauma) was based on the notion that one made psychological decisions about life at the time of birth. These decisions may become the basis for long-term living patterns that produce chronic inner conflict. For example, Orr (1977) felt that some common beliefs established at birth were that life is a struggle, the world is a dangerous place, or men hurt me (the male obstetrician who removed the infant with forceps and slapped the child into breathing was often the first contact with life). Although many of these approaches are based on the perhaps presumptuous notion that all birth is traumatic and that therefore each of us has a psychological disturbance right from the beginning of life, the fact that birth has for so long been acknowledged as a psychological event speaks to the profound emotional impact of child-bearing on each of us.

The Gestalt Approach to Birth

Whenever an event carries an emotional impact, resolution is required. For some, the act of being born may have been resolved instantaneously when the attending nurse washed and cared for the infant or when the child cried out at birth. For others, there may have been a tendency to relive some aspect of their own birth experience for the sake of resolving the event. Although we tend to relive our life scripts or dramas with similar roles, scenes, and characters, we do so out of an inner urge toward well-being. The psychological tendency to repeat past scenes that carry unresolved hurt or conflict is always an attempt to create an opportunity for personal healing. Samuels and Bennett, in *Be Well* (1974), described our tendency toward physical health. We have the same inner, life-giving drive toward mental health as well.

The Primal Therapist's Understanding

Arthur Janov (1971), in his work as a primal therapist, noted the tendency of clients to relive scenes regressively back to birth. He videotaped hundreds of primal patients re-experiencing their own birth for the purpose of present-day healing, and he noted relief of present-day problems through the release of birth-related emotion or psychical distress still held at the somatic level (in the body), such as the individuals who complained of chronic headaches. After resolving the forceps deliveries, the headaches disappeared. Janov's videotapes of men and women in the birth primal sound much like a woman in the final stages of labor pushing forth her child, with the magnificent gutteral sounds common to women who are allowed to express their feelings without interference of drugs or disapproval. One woman had always believed that the only things worth having in life were those that she had to work hard for. She labored for forty-two hours before her son was born. Her mother had labored equally long at the time of her own birth, in the same hospital where she was now delivering her son. Her belief that she had to work hard in order for things to have value might have led to the prolonged, painful labor. The tendency to relive her own birth for the purpose of resolution might have influenced her decision to give birth some three hundred feet from where she herself was born, a common decision among many women who find themselves drawn to the town or area where they themselves were born. This urge to return to the birth scene is expressed symbolically at Christmas each year and is also instinctive in the animal kingdom. Salmon, for instance, spawn and swim out to sea. After they reach maturity and are themselves ready to spawn, they swim upriver against great odds in order to lay their eggs. Biologists at the Salmon Fish Hatcheries on the Capilano River in British Columbia report that the salmon often lays her eggs within four inches of her own birthplace.

In the early 1970s, Arthur Janov and Frederick Leboyer appeared in public discussions of birthing practices. Leboyer (1975) said, "Dr. Janov and I have been following the same way. . . . I was trying to avoid what he was trying to make up for; he was trying to repair what had not been avoided." Janov (1971), noticing the tendency in women to relive their birth scenes, believed that every woman when giving birth was reliving her birth. The Mayan culture of Mexico has a postpartum custom that supports Janov's view. Brazelton, in *On Becoming a Family* (1981), reports that Mayan women are wrapped (swaddling style) in blankets, placed next to their infants, and cared for with the same special nurturing given to the infant. Similarly, certain Indian customs call for full-body massage of both mother and infant, as described by Leboyer in *Loving Hands* (1976). These postpartum care practices appear to create more rapid physical recovery in mothers and less prolonged psychological depression.

The Regressive-Recall Approach

There have been many studies in recent years using hypnosis with adults and simple recollection with children to recreate birth memories. In *Life before Life* (1979), Helen Wambach reported interviews with over seven hundred hypnotized subjects, with some 85 to 90 percent recalling actual birth memories. She used guided fantasy and suggestion without details. The subjects recalled life in utero, the journey through the birth canal, and entrance into the world. Linda Mathison, in "Down the Tunnel: An Inquiry into the Memories of the Very Young" (1980), describes two cases of clear recollection with children under 3 years of age. One child said, "I came down the tunnel. It was light. It was cold." The other said, "It's too tight. It's too bright. Daddy has a white coat on."

Whether or not one believes in the possibility of birth memories, the principal point is that one's birth has some effect on one's life. This effect may also result from, or be strengthened by, family stories about an individual's birth carried on as a favorite family joke or a dramatic story. A man named Paul recounted his story in a recent seminar; Paul was the tenth of eleven children born of farm parents. His mother gave birth to him at home on a rainy night in late March. The roads were thick with mud, and the doctor slid into a ditch on the way to the birth. His father drove down the road to find the doctor and help pull his car out to safety. The doctor arrived just in time to cut the cord and provide emotional relief to a concerned family. Paul loved hearing this story as a child because it seemed so exciting.

Interestingly, Paul says he owns a vehicle with four-wheel drive because he is always concerned about becoming stuck during inclement New England weather.

Our Own Birth Is Relived!

The tendency to relive unresolved birth experiences may also account for the strong need for mothering expressed by women during childbearing. Helene Deutsch noticed this need of women to be mothered. In *The Psychology of Women* (1945), she describes the inner urge to become dependent, perhaps in an effort to complete the maternal-child relationship. Lyn Delliquadri and Kati Breckenridge, in *Mother Care* (1977), say, "Passing from daughterhood to motherhood stirs up long-buried childhood memories and deeply felt needs for maternal warmth and security." They cite an example of a new mother who expressed this by saying, "More than anything else, I wanted to be rocked and held and put to bed wrapped in a soft warm blanket with a satin binding." Unfortunately, many women today ignore these inner needs for fear of losing independence, and thus deny themselves the opportunity for psychic healing. The more conscious we are of our feelings, the more opportunity we have for release and resolution. Childbearing provides a wealth of opportunity for resolution of the past that may pave the way for a more emotionally positive birth in the future. The following birth resolution assisted Judy to experience a more relaxed, normal delivery than might otherwise have been possible.

Judy's story

Judy came to us frightened that she would deliver her third child too fast. Her first child was born after a four-hour labor. The hospital personnel were not able to anticipate her birthing so rapidly and were unprepared. They madly rushed through the ordinary interferences—I.V., enema, prepping, etc.—leaving Judy with an especially acute sense of violation and lack of support.

Her second child was, again, a very fast delivery, creating a "mad dash" to the hospital and a fear that her child would be born en route. Her daughter was born in the hospital but had some breathing difficulties.

When Judy became pregnant for the third time, she came to us out of fear that her labor would be even faster and less supportive to her baby. In a recall processing session (a process of reliving past feelings for the purpose of emotional release), she remembered her own birth as a time of chaos and confusion and felt that everything was happening "too fast." When she checked with her mother, she was told that she "shot out like a cannonball." She also discovered that her father had been commissioned into the army and was leaving one day after her due date. He was constantly reminding her mother to "hurry up and give birth."

Once Judy discovered and released these memories and events, the fear of fast delivery disappeared. Her third child was born after a longer (six-hour), more relaxed labor in a hospital setting, supported by a kind and helpful medical team. She and her child were able to bond effectively.

Family Traditions

Each family has a heritage of beliefs and traditions about women and their roles. Some families, for example, describe women as "tough as nails" or "strong as oxen," referring to their ability to carry on under stress or difficulty. This usually refers to a woman's emotional or physical endurance capacities rather than her intellectual or business nature. Other cultural groups perceive women as weak or fragile and in need of protection and advice. Muriel James and Dorothy Jongeward, in *Born to Win* (1973), note that such script themes in the form of heritage and belief are carried on for years and greatly influence a woman's view of herself and the world around her. Extending this view to childbearing practices, women may hear messages such as, "The women in our family all have Cesareans or breeches."

Religious Beliefs and Childbearing

In considering the influences of family traditions on childbearing experiences, it is useful to include a review of religious influences. As far back as the Hindu medical writings (around 1400), male obstetrical specialists were called in to aid rich women in so-called complicated births. It would seem that the earliest interventions of the male in birth are associated with the abnormal or complicated deliveries. The Christian Biblical traditions speak of the woman who "travaileth in pain," suggesting great suffering and martyrdom in childbirth. The long-suffering sexless statues in Roman Catholic churches throughout the Western world certainly do not connote a woman in celebration of feminine sexuality. Birth is a sexual experience and our Christian religious influences have taught us to keep our legs closed, a condition that is not conducive to natural, positive birthing. In some religious traditions, menstruating women are refused participation in certain rituals, while others separate men and women, assuming uncleanliness in women.

It is difficult for us to rejoice in the ultimate celebration of our sexuality that is manifest in childbirth if our God-related images of women are neuter-gender, long-suffering martyrs (Blessed Virgin) or sinister seducers (Eve) who bring men to their downfall. Suzanne Arms (1975) writes that because Eve "ate of the apple," women were warned that they would be forevermore punished by their own bodies. According to the Bible, "I will greatly multiply thy sorrow and thy conception; in sorrow thou shalt bring forth children; and thy desire shall be to thy husband and he shall rule over thee" (Gen. 3:16). Perhaps our own mothers were influenced by this cursed command when they found themselves with five or more children and their own sense of well-being demanded fewer. The mind of a child is easily captured by information related in story form. Bandler and Grinder, in *The Structure of Magic* (1975), remind us of the power of the metaphorical statement over a more direct, nonmetaphorical statement. There is also an unconscious tendency to try to align oneself with religious or Godlike images in an attempt to insure some immortal reward after death. Far too many women, unaware of the teachings of early childbirth, may still be "travailing in birth" and "pained to be delivered" (Rev. 12:1, 2), bringing unnecessary suffering and emotional hurt upon themselves. How different many of us might have felt about our sexuality if the female statues were wearing low-cut dresses, shorter skirts, hands on hips, or just cracking a sexy smile. What relief!

One woman remembered that during a Christmas celebration at her family's church around her fifteenth year, she realized that the teaching of the day was that the Blessed *Virgin* was the *mother* of Jesus. Since her name was Mary Ann, she was particularly interested in the Virgin's activities. Not only was this a Virgin Mother, but she also had a nice man with a donkey taking care of her, apparently because she was "knocked up" at the time. That idea seemed quite appealing to Mary Ann, and has apparently appealed to many young Catholic women, judging by the statistics for Catholic unwed mothers. Just three years earlier, Mary Ann's mother had given birth to her fourth child by Cesarean section. Since it was a planned, repeat Cesarean, it appeared to be a "no-muss, no-fuss" birth. From this, combined with Christmas-card images that portrayed the Virgin Mother without labor pains or signs of delivery, Mary Ann concluded that Jesus was delivered in the same "no-muss, no-fuss" style as her brother and decided that childbirth did not require much involvement on the part of the mother.

Mothers Impress Daughters—The Family Legacy

Along with cultural influences, religious images and the familial legacy of the female, each woman forms her impressions of childbearing by listening to and observing the most important woman in her life: her own mother. As children, we even tend to absorb the feelings of our mothers, internalizing them as our own, in an attempt to help or relieve our mother's pain. Or, if we hear stories—such as that someone "nearly died in childbirth," "The women in our family have small pelvises," "Sex during pregnancy injures babies," "You lose a tooth for every baby," or "We all carry breech"— childbearing may become an expression of fear or a tradition of loyalty to a past that need not be repeated.

Nancy Cohen and Lois Estner (1983) remind us that our loyalties to our mother may be costing us greatly in unnecessary interventions and even surgical deliveries. This loyalty to childhood beliefs has nothing to do with loving our parents. Most psychotherapists would agree that the more re- leased we are from past connections and obligations, the more free we are to love in the present with respect for what has passed. Yet, as adults we still attempt to heal our parents by reenacting their lives.

"Scripted" into Pregnancy

Throughout this work, the notion of "script" has been discussed in order to illustrate the idea of repeated life patterns with recurring outcomes. Such recurrences were clearly indicated in the stories of fifteen unwed mothers, all members of the same support group organized by a family-planning clinic. The mothers ranged in age from 13 to 17 years. Of the fifteen, eleven had themselves been born to teenage mothers, out of wedlock, with absentee fathers. Nine of them were due to deliver their babies at exactly the same age their mothers were at the time the now-pregnant teenagers had been born. Most of them actually conceived their children under similar condi- tions to their own conception scene. The clearest example of "script" was demonstrated in the case of Michelle, a 15-year-old girl who had conceived her child in the back seat of her boyfriend's car on a hot night in August while parked in the back row of a drive-in movie theater. She remembered her mother telling her from about age 9 on that she should not go to the drive-in in the summer heat with her boyfriend. It was the best way for a girl to get pregnant. The thought was planted and the results produced.

Old Wives' Tales Become New Wives' Tales

Family traditions, often based on "old wives' tales" rather than healthful, positive childbearing practices, may be discussed among women even as adults and still carry a mental impact. Because of their reactivating quality, these tales may cause women to reinternalize the beliefs in the same childlike way of the past. Joann Bromberg, in "Having a Baby: A Story Essay" (1981), describes how the exchange of personal stories is a means of gathering information for childbearing women. She notes that "most speakers elabo- rated on bad experiences in some detail and referred only briefly to good ones." Perhaps Bromberg's study indicates a tendency for family members, too, to elaborate on the painful events rather than the joyful ones. Alice's story describes such a family tradition.

Alice's Story

Alice came for counseling after seven years of infertility. She was distraught and hopeless. She had not menstruated in two years and felt hopeless about the prospect of physical recovery. In tracing her history, it was discovered that seven years prior she had miscarried at almost five months. This experience had left her, as she described, "emotionally devastated."

When Alice became pregnant, she told only her mother and her husband about her pregnancy. Her mother, a usually strong influence in her life, told her that she should not tell anyone about her pregnancy before the fifth month because if she did she would suffer terrible embarrassment if she lost her child. Ordinarily, women are told that they should wait three months before sharing the news of their pregnancy, as though miscarriages are a terrible failure to be hidden from family and friends and handled in solitude.

In Alice's family, five months was considered the appropriate number. So, Alice waited until the middle of her fourth month, haunted by her mother's words of caution. She had an uneventful and healthy first trimester, supported by good medical reports. Finally, Alice became so excited and delighted with herself that she could not wait another day to share her good news. At a nephew's christening, she announced her pregnancy to all. The family was overjoyed, except for her mother, who stared with a disapproving glance.

The next morning, without warning, Alice miscarried while urinating. The scene was one of horror and disbelief. Alice was taken to the hospital, where she was essentially dusted off and sent home to get pregnant again. Her family tradition held true, and Alice was left with unresolved grief, fear, and feelings of failure.

Since processing out these events, Alice has begun to menstruate again. She reports a sense of balance and harmony in her physical body and renewed faith in its inner workings, and she can now reconsider her need or desire to have children based on her present life conditions.

Siblings' Births: A Part of Our Own Story

In addition to spoken words and familial beliefs, sibling births create a psychological impact. Until recently, there were very few, if any, pictorial accounts of childbirth suitable for children. Parents, burdened with a legacy of taboos on discussing sex, attempted to present their children with some explanation of pregnancy, childbirth, and the coming of a new sibling. Out of fear, embarrassment, and lack of tools, parents resorted to stories of birds and bees, storks, and angels. Although the stork legend was based on his tender, caring approach and his dwelling habits among watery places that were considered "soul" habitats, the explanation has rarely satisfied any sighted, intuitive Western child.

Mothers and fathers may be additionally suffering with fears of deserting children and not being able to manage another child with the necessary attention. T. Berry Brazelton (1981) describes an example of behavior changes in an 18-month-old, due in part to the mother's concerns about separation and also to the child's own innate ability to sense separation. He writes, "The more a woman cares for her child and the more she wants to do an ideal job with him (her), the more anguish she is likely to feel about deserting him and not being equal to the care of a second child."

Displaced Children

In this emotional upheaval, parents may find their own emotional expression and verbal communication difficult, so that pregnancy and childbirth are left to mystery and imaginations that may fill in the unknown with fearful, inaccurate beliefs.

Marcia's Story

One woman, Marcia, participating in a positive birthing seminar with a pregnant friend, burst into tears during the discussion of the sibling birth experience. She revealed that she was the oldest of seven children and that each time her mother became pregnant, Marcia lost a little more of her. Marcia remembered that her mother seemed embarrassed about discussing her pregnancies and mostly just ignored them. Marcia also sensed that her mother was angry, especially during the last three pregnancies. Marcia felt that this anger was due to her mother's not wanting to have more children, yet feeling blocked in her choice by her Roman Catholic beliefs about birth control. Marcia associated pregnancy with great emotional loss and separation from people you love. (It was interesting that she herself had had three miscarriages.)

Marcia cried because she had been trying to ease herself out of her friend Cathy's life, although she deeply loved Cathy and was genuinely excited by her pregnancy. Marcia felt that by separating herself from Cathy, she could protect herself from the unbearable separation she had felt as a child. Although Marcia might still have felt upset during her mother's pregnancy and birthing of her siblings, her inability to share her concerns, fears, and other emotions compounded a lonely time with further isolation. Incidentally, Marcia had very distant relationships with her last three siblings and felt toward them a resentment that she could not previously understand.

Some families are able to share feelings about sibling births. Although this process may not necessarily eliminate sibling rivalry, it may reduce the imagined scares of birth and the emotionally charged hurts that later can interfere with childbearing.

"Little Mommies and Daddies"

Occasionally, children are "prepped" with ideas about loving their siblings and feeling like little "mommies" and "daddies." This is only a partial approach to reality.

Children more often feel a full range of feelings toward siblings, such as Sharon's story describes. She writes:

I am forever grateful to my grandmother. I am the oldest of five children. For the first three years of my life, I was blissed out on parent and grandparent attention. I was the first grandchild and the apple of a lot of eyes. Then, a month after my third birthday, Lois was born. I was told how wonderful it would be to have company and to help take care of a baby. When my sister arrived home from the hospital, I did not think she was wonderful. I thought she was a nuisance, as she captured so much of the attention I once commanded. I began to have dreams of how I would open her bedroom window and find a giant green leaf. I dreamt that I placed her on the leaf and dropped her out the window so she could float gently to the ground. I felt bad about my dreams even though I never really pictured my sister injured or dead—just floating away.

When my second sister, Janice, was born two years later, I was more attuned to what was about to happen. I stayed at my grandmother's while my mother was in the hospital, which was rather long since Janice was an emergency Cesarean delivery. I started to cry one night and my grandmother, in her incredible wisdom, said that lots of children feel sad, mad, hurt, and scared when their mothers go to have babies. She said that she knew it was hard for me to have all this company even though I probably liked it sometimes. She said she knew I might not always feel like being nice to my sisters and that sometimes I might feel that my mother and father loved them more than me. I might even think that my parents forgot about me or did not care about me. She said I might wish I was a baby again and imagine myself drinking bottles and getting picked up on mom's shoulder. My grandmother went on to say that all these feelings were okay and that I would probably notice I also had some good, happy feelings too. She said God loved me no matter what I thought or felt and so did she.

After these moments with her, I felt whole and good again. The recurring dream about my sister Lois disappeared. I still was not completely fond of having to share all those wonderful adults in my life, but I felt better about meeting my new sister. Childbirth, instead of causing me hurt and fear, now seemed more okay. Pregnancy was still a well-kept secret, but it didn't seem so painful after that.

Adolescent Sexuality and Body Images

All of us, men and women alike, collect data about sex, pregnancy, birth, and bodies during our adolescent years. Helene Deutsch (1945) has likened childbearing to adolescence in that we are once again faced with bodily changes, functional differences, and emotions related to sexuality. This reactivation of adolescent fears, embarrassment, guilt, or inadequacy may influence a woman's psychological approach to childbirth as well as a man's. Men in childbearing will be discussed in a future chapter. Here, the focus will be on the influence of adolescent sexuality and body image on the childbearing process in women.

Body Acceptance/Body Rejection

In the adolescent years, women are particularly subject to body acceptance or rejection, and we may learn at that time to associate feelings of shame and embarrassment with our own bodies and others' bodies. As infants, parents pat us on the back and praise us for burping, cheer us for defecating, and giggle when we pass gas. Infants lie in the middle of a room naked while surrounding adults admire the beauty and innocence of a child's body.

Then, one day we burp and someone calls us a pig, or we pass some gas and everyone says, "Phew!" When we defecate, they tell us to hurry and flush it, and if we take off our clothes for some of that old admiration, somebody asks, "Where's your modesty?"

Sometime between the ages of 9 and 13, young girls discover that anything that is not destined to become a 34B size 9 is unacceptable. We learn to use deodorant and perfumes to cover our smells and make-up to cover our faces. Pimples become unacceptable imperfections along with perceived or actual excess body fat.

SEX: The Forbidden Subject

Sex and sexual parts may be discussed, but often in an attitude of moral repressiveness. Menstruation may be a source of fear and embarrassment, especially since girls are often told that sanitary napkins are objects to be hidden (further supported by the druggist, who hurries to cover the box with a paper bag before taking your money). In some religions, women are even today refused certain rituals during menstruation, as they are seen as unfit at this time. Nancy Friday, in *My Mother, My Self* (1978), writes, "My friends and I knew all about those blue and white Kotex boxes in our mothers' bathrooms. . . . Beginning menstruation meant two things to me: relief that it wasn't appendicitis and deep embarrassment at having to go through the initiation rites with my mother."

As we physically developed our sexual bodies, the development of breasts and hips often served as signals for fathers with daughters to back off and cease physical contact. For young girls whose fathers had been quite affectionate, this restraint usually came as quite a shock and activated feelings of rejection and hurt in association with the physical, sexual body. This is particularly true in families that did not discuss these events verbally and therefore left much room for a young teenage girl's imagination to create reasons for the rejection.

Most women, as teenagers, were taught to sexually control themselves at all times regardless of circumstances or desires. We usually waited to become biology students before fully understanding our physical beings, and even then most of us only got to see the sexual parts of a frog.

The Body's Beauty Reclaimed!!

Delliquadri and Breckenridge, in *Mother Care* (1979), write, "If you are like most women, you have probably been critical of your body since the onset of puberty; this may influence your experience in getting used to your pregnant and post-partum body."

How difficult for women to accept the fact that extra body weight may be necessary to nourish and produce healthy babies, when women have been programmed to fear every ounce beyond a size 9 figure! How are we to welcome the rush of waters that preserved our child's life and the release of blood from the uterus that provided the food and nourishment for the walls of the protective womb? How are we to marvel at the miracle of the placenta when we were horrified at a mere pimple? We seek to give birth naturally, yet find disapproval even for the loud, "unladylike" sounds common to pushing stages.

Childbearing offers women an opportunity to release negative beliefs about the body that are not supportive to maternal well-being. Gayle Peterson, in *Birthing Normally* (1981), discusses how negative body beliefs and images lower a woman's self-esteem and cause her to feel weak and frail and to lose faith in her physical capacities, all of which negatively affect childbearing.

The physiology offered in childbirth education and preparation courses greatly aids in acceptance and understanding of the inevitable changes in the physical body, but only through emotional, heart-felt, self-love can the wonders of childbearing be fully appreciated and celebrated. The next story speaks to this point.

Joan's Story

Joan, a 27-year-old attorney, came in in the third month of her second pregnancy. Her first child had been born three years previously after a long, difficult labor that resulted in a Cesarean delivery. She was convinced that her body had not functioned effectively due to some emotional blocks, since her pelvis measured sufficiently (although pelvic size is usually irrelevant) and there were no signs of fetal distress. The Cesarean birth was encouraged because Joan had apparently reached a state of physical and emotional exhaustion.

In tracing her history, it was discovered that her first love-making scene was very painful to her. She was 17 at the time, and had been going steady with the same boy for three years. After restraining themselves for years, they finally decided to have sex—convincing themselves in the 1960s style that they would be married someday so that any wrongdoing would right itself.

One evening when her parents were at work, Joan and her boyfriend went to her bedroom to have sex. In the middle of their passion, her father came home and found her and her boyfriend. In a rage, he called her a slut and a whore, and told her that her body was just a "piece of junk." He dragged her off to the local minister, who confirmed these views and demanded that she never again "open herself" to "sexual contacts"—he even forgot to say "unless she was married."

Joan was completely humiliated and lived in shame for months afterwards. Pressured by her father and the minister, she broke up with her boyfriend. She felt isolated, embarrassed, and irredeemable. Joan was able to release the pain of these events and become more loving toward her body. Her second baby was born vaginally after a normal, effective, eight-hour labor, an experience that Joan describes as a celebration of herself.

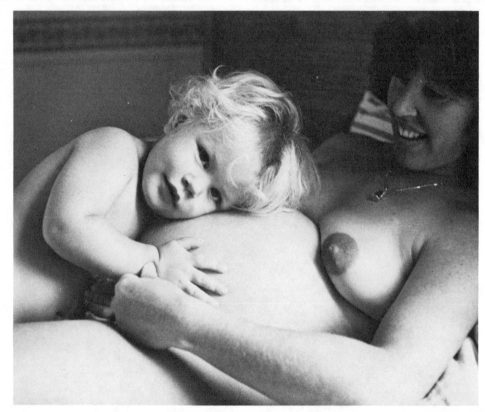

©Jackie Murphy-Knapp

5

Clearing Past Pregnancy and Childbirth Experiences

In 1982, approximately 3.5 million American women gave birth (Bureau of Natality 1980). Some of these women experienced the joy and miracle of childbearing. They celebrated these births with self-affirmation, pride, and appreciation for their own strengths and resources. They will recall childbirth with inner confidence and faith in their physical bodies. They will have begun the all-important maternal-child relationship with a strong foundation of harmony, reflected in their personal feelings about birth and their inner pride at having successfully managed a highly stressful event. We celebrate you all!

There are many, perhaps millions, of women who may feel the aforementioned joy and pride, but may also feel guilty, inadequate, weak, and vulnerable, and may define themselves as failures. Their birthing experiences may become a source of inner hurt or outward resentment for many years to come. Their children, although deeply loved, may also become symbols of self-hate, failure, or inadequacy. The normal stress of childbearing may become distress and family conflict in the future. We celebrate you all and pray that you remain conscious and aware of these feelings until they are completely released and replaced by natural joy and self-love.

Of the 3.5 million birthing women, all of them grieved—some with great respect for the psychological necessity and accompanying emotions, others in unconscious, unaware states of hurt, loneliness, and fear.

Furthermore, somewhere between 700,000 and 800,000 women were surgically delivered and faced the awesome task of post-operative as well

53

as postpartum recovery. Almost 200,000 women gave birth to lifeless children and spent many months grieving and hurting without anywhere near the necessary support. Finally, another 35,000 to 40,000 women gave birth to children who died within a day or a week, leaving their parents to remember their cries or eyes or some small movement for the rest of their lives (Peppers & Knapp 1980). These are not happy thoughts, and they do not support our fairy-tale approaches to childbearing. Not one of these parents—and there were more than a million of them—sat in childbirth preparation courses believing that this could happen to them.

The impact of Cesarean delivery and/or fetal and infant loss is profound, and the psychological realities and necessary supports will be discussed in future chapters. Here, we are discussing the psychological impact of past experiences, with a major focus on normal, vaginal birthing.

Past Pregnancies and Births: Impact Present and Future

Past pregnancy and childbirth experiences lay the foundation for future births and therefore greatly influence birthing outcomes. Sheila Kitzinger (1981) writes that when women have suffered some inner hurt or humiliation in childbearing, this experience affects their whole lives, including the maternal-child relationship and relationships with other birthing women. Gayle Peterson, in *Birthing Normally* (1981), explains how she uses slides of positive birth outcomes to help women view birth in a positive way rather than as a reflection of some past experience that does not support a positive outcome now. Others in the field, such as Nancy Cohen, coauthor of *Silent Knife*, have also realized the importance of previous experiences and devote several sessions of VBAC preparation to clearing past violations and hurts (Cohen & Estner 1983).

Repeating the Past in Attempts to Heal Past Hurt

As discussed in an earlier chapter, there is an unconscious tendency to repeat any unresolved past events in an attempt to release inner hurt and achieve psychological resolution. This was obvious, perhaps, in the stories of the unwed mothers who themselves had been born out of wedlock. This tendency to seek repetition, as well as the mental resistence to change, often leads women to repeat previous experiences at the emotional and sometimes even the physical level. The physical manifestation of leftover hurt and conflict is probably most often experienced as a result of a lack of faith in one's body, combined with a self-fulfilling prophecy that the body is not working right. Ellen's story expresses this lack of faith and resulting outcome.

Ellen's Story

Ellen was a 34-year-old woman who had delivered her first child, Katie, by Cesarean a year earlier. Ellen was still experiencing anger, fear, help-lessness, and sadness about the events of Katie's birth. She was particularly burdened with feelings of anger and hatred toward her doctor, her husband, and, most especially, her older sister. She also experienced physical pain in the edges of the Cesarean scar, which she felt reflected how she was feeling about the birth and her body. She recalled that throughout her childhood she had felt that her sister and her mother discounted her fem-ininity and generally undermined her self-confidence. Ellen viewed her sister as a model daughter and a model student, who seemed to do everything perfectly. Ellen viewed herself, on the other hand, as incompetent and inept, and now saw herself as having a body that did not work.

During her labor with Katie, Ellen was able to dilate to 7 centimeters quite successfully. Then, all further dilation ceased. After hours of ineffective labor, Ellen was exhausted and agreed to a Cesarean. Ellen's history revealed two miscarriages prior to her Cesarean delivery, both of which reinforced her view that her body did not function properly. After several counseling sessions, Ellen was able to understand how her anger toward herself de-bilitated her physical capacities; she next sought to release herself from her lack of faith in her body. Through the use of positive mental imagery, she healed her Cesarean scar, and she began to gain faith in her body's capacities to heal and to seek well-being.

Resolving the Past:
A Resource for Our Future

Previous childbirth experiences also serve to establish our capacities to manage the stress of pregnancy, labor, birth, and postpartum. Seminar attendants have reported this phenomenon in two common ways, although there are as many styles as there are women.

Let Go of Hurt—Stop Being the Victim

First, there are those women who experienced feelings of hurt, anger, fear, resentment, guilt, and so on in childbearing, feelings that were inter-nalized as a sign of weakness, inadequacy, and, in some cases, pathology. These women tend to harbor an inner fear of repetition of the same and an attitude of being beaten before they start.

Second, there are those women who experienced upset in childbirth and externalized the experience, feeling angry and violated by the system. Out of this outward anger and inner humiliation, these women perceive child-birth as another chance to prove they can do it, prove they can fight the system. These women tend to carry an "I'll show them" attitude.

Neither of these positions supports maternal well-being. They are both paths to increased likelihood of further failure—one out of feeling powerless, the other out of feeling falsely powerful without a genuine resolution of past hurt. Childbearing should be neither a psychological catastrophe nor a po-litical battlefield. Recognizing and releasing pregnancy- and birth-related upsets creates a calm mind, a relaxed body, and an emotional system that is open for new experiences. Transactional analysis theory describes mental filing systems of emotional experiences as stamp collecting (Berne 1972). Each time one experiences an event of similar emotion, a trading stamp is added to the stamp book that contains that particular emotion, such as anger or fear. When the stampbook or emotional stack is full, one feels justified in redeeming the collected books. A book is full when there is no psycho-logical space to contain the emotion, e.g., anger, without releasing enough to clear a page in the book. A common Western expression for this phe-nomenon is "the straw that broke the camel's back."

Past pregnancy and childbirth experiences may have so much unreleased emotion attached to them that a woman finds herself overwhelmed with feelings in the present pregnancy or birth experience. Experiences that might otherwise have resulted in a minor upset and might be normal stress-related events may become the final stamp in the psychological collection, the stamp that "breaks the camel's back." Women do not need to enter present-day birth experiences with the emotional burden of past events. Good information and adequate support can alleviate this unnecessary added stress.

Release through the Written Word

Clearing oneself of the past may take many forms, ranging from sharing with a friend to writing series of letters. Here are some letters that were written for release and healing. Some were mailed, some were not. We now carry to our seminars a trash can complete with furry, green Oscar the Grouch. Oscar, as we already know, eats pizza with bananas, mudpies, and broken toys, and loves stinkweed. He also eats unwanted papers, feelings, and thoughts, and gladly accepts all donations from anyone who has past birth-related hurts that need a place to go. These donations were made to Oscar. They were written for release, not for blame. They were written to express unwanted feelings and are only truly complete when forgiveness and peace of mind are achieved.

Dear Dr. M.,

Sharon is growing so rapidly—and so beautifully—that I almost can't envision what she looked like at birth. Almost...no, that's not nearly true, for everything about her birth is still crystal clear and "alive" to me. What a joy it was to have a daughter! Her tiny, strong body; her bright and wide-open eyes searching into mine; her fingers closing around my thumb—all these images are engraved on my heart. I remember turning to you, Dr. M., choking with emotion, and thanking you. In that moment I felt so "beholden" to you, so aware of your role at Sharon's birth. Yet, something was not quite right. Some sadness and regret tinged my joy, and I couldn't dispel those feelings. Time passed, and my sadness grew, no matter how I tried to heal it with gratitude for my healthy baby. Now I feel compelled to express my feelings to you, partly because I think—and hope—that you care about doing your job well and partly because I care about the women and babies who will come after me, and mostly because I need to do so. I felt robbed at Sharon's birth. Cheated. Manipulated. Ripped off. Something terribly important was missing, and I felt its loss. At first, I couldn't explain what was gone, but suddenly I knew: it was me. At first, there I was, laboring to birth my first child, awed by the miracle of life within me. For most of my labor, my husband and I had worked hard together, alone, and we did just fine. I felt soaring pride in us, and I felt amazed by my own strength. But then, suddenly, when labor speeded up and birth seemed close, you took over. **You took over.** Do you know what that means?? You took away my right to give birth and gave me instead a delivery. You took away my autonomy, my sense that I was birthing my child, and made me a little girl doing what "Doctor M." decreed. You covered my body with green sheets, you tied down my arms, you took away my power and strength. I was forced to lie passively and uncomfortably, to push at your command. Don't you know that pushing while lying flat is pushing uphill—and when I felt that resistance, that denial of nature, you told me to relax, that you'd take care of everything. Well, I wanted to take care of everything. And then, when my uphill pushing wasn't effective, you sliced open my perineum so you could deliver my baby.

I can't blame you totally for displacing me, for I abdicated my right to give birth. I would have done anything to protect my baby, and then I thought you should know best how to safeguard her. Now I know better. Now I know that she would have been even safer had I followed my instincts, my deep body knowledge of how to give birth. Mothers know that best, and excepting rare emergencies, doctors should be there not to usurp maternal instinct, but to support and strengthen it.

One last thing. After Sharon was born, as I lay laughing and crying and hugging Bill, you told me to slow down my breathing. "If you don't, you'll get dizzy," you said, "and I can't stand dizzy women." I felt dishonored and categorized with all the other "dizzy women" you've disserved. In truth, Dr. M., we aren't dizzy at all. We feel strong, invincible, limitless surges of love for our babies, and we feel pride in the strength and power of our bodies. We want that love and power respected and honored, not *strapped down, or sliced apart, or covered with ugly green sheets. And most of all, we—I—want to **give birth**, not be delivered. Could you stand by and watch the miracle of birth? Would your ego survive? I pray that you could and will, for to give birth is a woman's inherent right. Please don't dismiss or take it lightly; the courage and faith and strength of countless women through the ages waits to be upheld.*

It's not easy to think of forgiving you, but I know that if I hold this anger I will remain forever powerless.

B.D.

Dear Dr. O.,

I am writing this letter to you out of concern for my mental well-being. . . .

Let us start from the beginning (October 1981) when I had need of your services under what I felt were emergency circumstances. . . . I was bleeding abnormally for some time with no apparent reason. I had missed my period for one week. I suspected a pregnancy although you initially discounted this assumption because I had no breast tenderness and didn't "feel pregnant." When I asked why I shouldn't have a pregnancy test you replied, "There is no sense in complicating the picture with extraneous testing at this time. Your bleeding will stop in a few days." Dr. O., why in hell didn't you listen to what you were hearing? You have taken such a "holier-than-thou" attitude about your technical capabilities and have failed to look at the humanistic side of things. . . . I feel that my case was mismanaged. Perhaps an earlier diagnosis would have saved my right Fallopian tube? You know damn well that it would have. . .Eight days later I was still bleeding. You immediately ordered a pregnancy test. I waited—positive. You ordered an ultrasound. Results: a mass on the right side. No uterine pregnancy. And you still filled me with false hope. "It could be an ovarian cyst, you may have miscarried already." No need to worry. "We'll do a laparoscopy tomorrow and depending on the results you may or may not have a tube when you wake up from the anesthesia." I thought, "You bastard. You are so goddamn quick to get me to that operating room. Why weren't you as quick in picking up the diagnosis earlier?"

Needless to say, I was devastated when I came out of the anesthesia. . . . And where were you? It will be a while before I can forgive.

L.P.

Dear Dr. Y.,

It has been five years since you delivered my daughter. As I look back on the events of her birth, I feel upset and very resentful when I see your face and hear your voice in my mind.

I remember when we had our eighth-month appointment about what kind of anesthesia I would have. I told you then that I wanted natural childbirth with no medication. You were not supportive at all, you said that giving birth was really painful and I should think about it more. But if I was determined I would have to take the childbirth course at the hospital before you would consider it.

The day came. I came to the hospital in the morning. Before I was even examined I was given an enema. I had never had an enema, so I had no idea of what to expect. I had heard people say that enemas were awful, so when I was sitting on the toilet and I started having very strong cramping and pushing sensations, I thought it was because of the enema. When I realized the baby was almost here, I ran down the hall and you got me into the delivery room fast. My husband was told to hurry up and get into the white coverups or he would miss the delivery.

Instead of letting me go with the contractions and push like my entire body was doing, you made me hold my legs together and you said, "Don't push, we're not ready yet." My baby and I were ready! I had to fight against all the natural responses of my body so the anesthesiologist could put a needle in my spine and so that you could give me an episiotomy. When I moaned because it was so difficult not to push, I heard you say, "See, I told you natural childbirth was painful; the spinal will take effect soon."

You were right. Very soon I felt nothing. From the mirrors above me I saw you put your hand inside me, water came out and then my baby. You were so surprised. You didn't expect her so quickly.

I had to lie flat on my back for many hours after delivery without my baby because of a spinal that was not needed.

When I saw you the next day and you said, "Boy, that was fast," I told you the next baby I would have at home and bring the baby in with me. You laughed and said, "Oh no, we will be prepared for the next one, we will have you in here in plenty of time."

Dr. Y., I pray that you have changed your attitude about women not being capable of birthing their children. When I have another child, I will birth my child at home with people who are willing to be around to assist only in case of an emergency. I will push my baby into this world naturally and lovingly. I'm sorry for both of us.

D.K.

Celebrations—Let's Do More!

In addition to these expressions of disappointment, hurt, guilt, anger, etc., it is important to also include letters of celebration. There is a tendency in Western culture to dwell upon the negative. Don Dinkmeyer and Lewis E. Losconcy, in *The Encouragement Book* (1980), remind us that pain and suffering are perpetuated by negative thinking, and that discouragement ensues when all energy is focused on the painful side of life. This does not mean that we should support fairy-tale views of easy, painless childbirth or unconscious states of withheld feelings, but rather that birth as a celebration deserves equal time.

Madeleine Kenefick, in *Positively Pregnant* (1981), writes, "I spent a lot of time talking to women about their pregnancies. Very few had anything positive to say about the experience." Her book is written out of her belief that it is possible for women to "relish" rather than just "endure" their pregnancies. Although positive stories do not make good soap-opera material, they do make for a sound psychological basis for childbearing, especially after past upsetting feelings have been cleared.

Nancy Cohen, co-author of *Silent Knife*, has a delightful approach to birth as a celebration. She always brings party hats for everyone (including attending physicians) as a reminder that childbirth is somebody's birthday (Cohen & Estner 1983).

Letters for Joy and Self-Affirmation

Dear Anybody-Who-Wants-To-Hear,

Joy to the world! I did it. . . .I mean I really did it!! Jillian has been born. There isn't one thing about her birth that I would change—except maybe to have shared it with a few more good friends of mine. It was such a gift to John (my husband) and me—and I'd really like people to know about it so that they'd know what birthing really was about for me and how things can be.

It's amazing, too, because five months before her birth I really didn't believe I was capable of creating that type of experience. . . . Oh, what the love and support of friends can do! What screwed me up was fear and ignorance and machines and negative thoughts and lack of faith in my body and spirit. I learned to love myself and believe in myself and surround myself with people who feel the same. And I learned about what was going to physically happen to me and my baby so I could "go" with my labor. I knew I was going to work hard and that it was going to hurt sometimes, but that it was healthy pain and good work. I kept the machines away and didn't let anyone interfere with me and my baby unless I said it was okay and really knew it was necessary.

Originally, I was going to take my "show," at the last possible minute, to the hospital because my husband John just couldn't seem to make that final commitment to staying home. My doctor had promised that I could "do my thing" there and that our midwife could be the one to help me deliver our baby. But when I was actually in labor, John knew in his heart that home was where we belonged and he wholeheartedly committed to it. We had all the supplies and our midwife knew we knew what we were doing and were really prepared, so she said, "Great!". . . .

It was so wonderful to be in labor, totally surrounded by only love and positive support. Every birthing woman should know that feeling! And the total freedom I had to do whatever I wanted whenever I wanted was just terrific! Even little Adam (my son) was a source of comfort and joy. . . .

No matter when I had a contraction, someone seemed to know and was right there to touch me or massage me in just the right spot. When I wanted to walk I did, when I wanted to kneel over the bed, or stand or lie down, I did. When I wanted to curse a contraction I did and when I wanted to crack a joke, I had a great captive audience that really laughed. You know, it's really true that a relaxed, smiling mouth opens the vagina!

For a while I chose to labor in a warm bath and that was great. Boy, there's something about a hot tub. . . . The hot compresses to the perineum and the massage with vitamin E oil were both soothing and so helpful to the stretching process needed for birthing. I had it all.

The communication shared by John and me through touch, and word, and just with our eyes was magic. . . .

And when it came to pushing. . . .I chose to squat, with either one of the midwives or my friend Cathy sitting on the edge of the bed supporting me, and John at my feet with (the other midwife) ready for the baby. The hardest part of that was first pushing out this huge bag of forewaters. Once that was done it was only a matter of minutes.

. . .Our new baby was a beautiful, healthy girl!

. . .Is there anything better than a room bursting with love. . .into which to welcome your new baby?

L.L.

Dear World,

Thank you for giving me the opportunity to acknowledge myself and the clearing work I did so that I really got a decent birth experience.

Represented in our work was locating an excellent obstetrician. His support of me in having the birth the way I wanted it was a priority. . . .

I went in for an appointment with Dr. Z., who said I would be delivering in a few hours and I was to have the midwife drive me up right then. I believed he was being dramatic, as I felt nothing, but trusted his experience.

An hour later I was sitting in the birthing room with my midwife and my husband Sandy. . . . [After another hour, my] water broke [and] I was plunged into wall-like contractions that started from a peak and seemed to last a long time. No build up. I was being overtaken by a volcano or a hurricane. The breathing patterns that I had used for my other births clearly didn't work.

I had worked on the issue of breathing into the uterus, rather than attempting to avoid the pelvic region which seems to me what . . . [some others] do. My other two births were long, with complications. A lot of vomiting and sleepiness which today I view as my attempt to leave the scene.

I placed my attention in the uterus. . . . There was a shift in consciousness and I was crystal clear of my uterus and the baby within. We were in communication. I saw that any resistance on my part would [make] it harder and longer for her. I set the clear intention to open and let this being come in as easily as possible. . . .

We were all clear on our job. We were a unit, a family working in harmony. . . .

One of the beautiful aspects of Dr. Z. is he becomes the process. He is able to create himself with the woman in labor. He is not an intrusion. . . .

Katie was coming down fast and it hurt. I yelled, and Dr. Z., in total support of my intention to have a peaceful birth, told me to be quiet so I would not hurt her ears. It snapped me back to my job. He quieted the staff that was now full in the room, and lowered the lights. I forever love Dr. Z. for just doing his job. He invited Sandy to receive Katie so Sandy did!. . . .

Dr. Z. didn't cut the cord until she was breathing on her own. Sandy got to hold her. I delivered the placenta and the birth team left as soon as possible, letting Sandy, Katie and me bond. . .together in that perfect love. . . .

D.S.

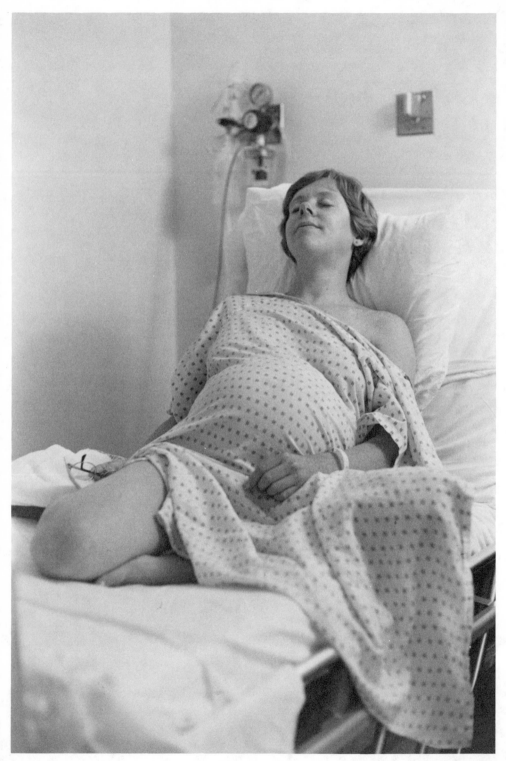

6

Pain, Politics, Power: Three Psychological Biggies

Pain

There has probably never been a Western childbearing woman who has not dreaded the pain of labor or hoped for a fast, painless delivery. Most women in our seminars, when asked what books they read prior to birth, proclaim *Painless Childbirth* (Lamaze 1958) as their first purchase. Certainly, we would all like to find a method that would avoid or elude pain. However, there are none.

There are, however, psychological states that promote and prolong pain, and there are conditions that decrease and transform pain. These psychological states can be altered by beliefs, attitudes, environments, support teams, and historical experiences of pain unique to each individual reality. Creating an optimum mental state is a realistic possibility for every childbearing woman.

Natural Childbirth: The American Myth

Genuine natural childbirth, although not synonymous with positive birthing, supports maternal and infant well-being and therefore serves as a useful goal whenever possible. It is estimated that between 90 and 96 percent of all births could be natural if properly supported, leaving only 4 to 10 percent of births requiring actual interventions (Mendelsohn 1981). Natural childbirth supports maternal well-being because it builds psychic resources and self-confidence, but more basically, natural childbirth eliminates interventional risks. Drugs are simply not safe and therefore must be used cautiously and from a position of informed choice. Natural childbirth is not just simply a psychological and physical challenge. It is not supported as an athletic event for performing entrants or an endurance test for pain tolerance. Natural childbirth is the *safest* approach to childbirth and therefore deserves careful consideration.

Try Hugs before Drugs

There are volumes of studies on drug usage during pregnancy, labor, and delivery and they all add up to the same conclusion, summed up by the Committee on Drugs of the American Academy of Pediatrics: "There is no drug, whether over-the-counter remedy or prescription drug, that, when taken or administered to a childbearing woman, has been proven safe for the child." Yet, it is estimated that 90 percent of all pregnant women take drugs, with an average of 4.5 drugs per mother (Arms 1975).

We know well the European tragedy of the Thalidomide babies of the 1950s, and the young women cancer patients whose mothers took DES in the 1950s and 1960s. We can read for ourselves the work of Dr. Alan Guttmacher, in *Pregnancy, Birth, and Family Planning* (1973), and Dr. Yvonne Brackbill (1974), who states, "The major obstetrical danger may now be medication itself." These writers speak to the dangers and compromises to the fetus inherent in *any* medication—from aspirin to paracervical block. As Suzanne Arms (1975) writes, "How many times must it be said? Drugs get to the baby. Drugs adversely affect the baby. Drugs may permanently damage the baby." So, natural childbirth is at least safe childbirth, unless (as happens relatively rarely) complications occur.

Although a review of the literature clearly assesses all drugs as potentially dangerous, a large number of women will be medicated during birth, not because they wish to risk injury or because doctors want to damage babies, but rather because childbearing women and men have not been given the psychological tools for maintaining psychological states conducive to pain reduction and transformation. Nor have physicians been trained in a total, holistic approach to medicine.

Pain Avoidance: The Path to UNNATURAL Childbirth

There are many approaches to pain. Fairy-tale approaches to childbearing (God knows we all like to believe in the painless-childbirth fairy tale) still refer to pain as "discomfort" or muscle tension. The idea behind this approach is to attempt to trick the mind into believing that the body need not be in pain and, therefore, it will not be. It is true that pain has cultural influences determined by one's mental state and accompanying beliefs. Dick-Read (1944) attempted to work with culturally induced pain caused by fear generated out of frightening stories of childbearing experiences passed on among women. It is also true that positive attitudes about childbearing produce positive results. In his study on "The Importance of Belief in the Childbearing Process" (1979), Lewis Mehl, M.D. predicted birthing outcomes with remarkable accuracy. His predictions were based on maternal mind sets. However, a particular breathing technique or physical exercise usually does not eliminate pain, and both are deceptive. Further, approaches that rely solely on positive thoughts for positive results also fail to adequately prepare women for the reality of physical pain common to most labors in Western cultures.

There are different approaches to and expressions of pain among cultures of the world. The Western approach to pain tends to be one of avoidance and association with medical need and illness, whereas other cultures have more acceptance and less stress. Brigitte Jordan, in *Birth in Four Cultures* (1980), described Mayan women in childbirth. She noticed an acceptance of pain among birth attendants, as if pain was simply taken for granted. The Kahuna men and women of Hawaii knew ways of giving pain to someone else who might be a lazy relative or someone considered deserving of the pain. Kahunas report "painless" labors while the unsuspecting relative groans and moans through the labor (Meltzer 1981). The Kahuna tribe demonstrates mastery of the mind in a form that is beyond Western comprehension but gives an example of ultimate mind control to the point of thought transference.

If Western women practiced meditation and mind control for many years, they might gain such control. The Masters of India who do not eat or drink for days beyond the expected survival period and Kahuna tribesmen who walk on hot coals prove the power of mind over matter. The American woman, flooded with external stimuli daily, will not likely gain such body mastery after only six or ten sessions of childbirth preparation.

Gayle Peterson (1981) writes that "not to effectively deal with the notion and experience of pain is to do a great disservice to women." She reminds us that pain is not all cultural and psychological in its nature and describes how this discomfort (pain) is not all in our heads. Attitudes and information affect the intensity and degree of pain as well as one's ability to effectively cope, but pain is still pain.

Beliefs Affect Degree of Pain

Attitudes and beliefs about pain and pain management influence birth outcomes. For example, as women, we have been trained to approach pain as damsels in distress, ridden with inner helplessness and in search of a handsome prince, or as overcompensating superwomen who can bring home the bacon, fry it up in the pan, and never let anyone know how tough it really is. In Chapter Four, the common psychological scripts or life dramas of many Western women were reviewed. Cinderella, Sleeping Beauty and Snow White were not known for their own personal resources, but rather confronted difficulty with nonconsciousness and helplessness. They were not models of psychological resource and competence.

Expectations of Failure

Teachings that approach pain as discomfort expect women to be incapable of handling it. Women who respond to accurate presentations of pain in labor with unconscious spacing out, actively discount their own ability to effectively cope with pain. Further, these approaches acutally increase pain by teaching avoidance, control, resistance, and endurance, rather than acceptance and surrender.

In our positive birthing seminars, women are invited to imagine that they are men—pregnant men. There is a wide variation in reported experiences, but the majority tend to report a different feeling and attitude associated with pain. As pregnant men, they often report a newfound sense of power. They realize that men would not have to bring their wives along to the obstetrician in order to get their questions answered. Some imagine they would not have to work so hard at practicing breathing exercises because as men they would be expected to effectively manage pain. Men are expected to train for, run, and complete marathons. Women are expected to take the event less seriously and may even be defined as eccentric for wanting to run in the first place. Football players are expected to go on with the game regardless of pain and without dramatization. Women are expected to stay off the football field and not to engage in such unlady-like activity. We would hardly expect to treat a pregnant man in the midst of labor as a damsel-in-distress.

In "Taking Care of the Little Woman" (1981), Coleman Romalis describes physician-father interactions, noting how the physician may attempt to bring the father into psychological collusion in order to "big daddy" the pregnant or birthing woman. Yet, we would not expect our obstetrician to refer to our husbands and male partners as the "little man." These attitudes do not support a woman's innate capacity for pain management.

Suzanne Arms, in *Immaculate Deception* (1975), describes how childbirth preparation courses are sometimes based on expectations of failure. She reminds us that hospital settings are designed in preparation for the woman to fail when relying entirely on her own resources; these settings suggest to birthing women that they need not worry about any coping difficulties, as they can be easily managed with interventions—despite the fact that most interventions have inherent risks. Further, since most women expect to have completely natural births (even though statistics show that only about 10 percent or less of American women actually birth naturally in hospital settings), women are confused about what constitutes a genuine crisis requiring intervention and what is actually a discount of their innate strength and capacity.

Reframing Pain: New Meaning in Childbirth

Some approaches attempt to reframe both the word "pain" and the accompanying experience. There is a certain usefulness in these procedures in that "pain" has been generally associated with illness, disease, emergency, injury, death, and general fear. Dictionary definitions include, "The unpleasant sensation of feeling resulting from or accompanying a physical injury, over-strain or disorder." Such descriptions do not include the words "natural" or "healthy"; they do not sound at all like Ina May Gaskin's term "energy rush" (1977). For many women, "pain" is associated with trauma, fear, and death. When asked what mental associations participants had with the word "pain," the following list was compiled:

"ouch"	hurt	infections
falling down	trauma	serious illness
death	terror	disease
hospitals	cuts	critical
dentistry	bleeding	intensive care
broken bones	doctors	aspirin
hot stoves	stitches	wine
drugs	earaches	avoid

None of these mental associations is conducive to relaxation and transformation of pain. When asked for a new mindset for childbirth pain, participants wrote:

moving	baby	arrival
surrender	rush	alive
gain	work	support
contraction	energy	help
birth	delivery	health

Normal Fear: A Sign of Mental Health

One of the greatest contributions of early childbirth educators, such as Dick-Read, Lamaze, and others, was the creation of a curriculum that would provide a sound understanding of the actual physiology of pregnancy, labor, and delivery. As the human mind has a tendency to fill in the "unknown" with probable or possible negative outcomes, informed childbearing greatly reduces the mind's tendency toward the frightful. When the mind is calm and knowledgeable about ongoing events, the body responds with like calm, a condition conducive to natural and more enlightened childbearing. Knowledge has the effect of decreasing fear and therefore pain.

In women with personal histories that abound with physical pain, birth-related pain may become another straw that breaks the camel's back, and therefore may need attention prior to birth. We have discussed the idea of psychological stacks that are reflections of similar experiences with like results. Pain stacks for some women may be full and easily activated. Understanding and releasing some of the emotional charge associated with these memories can be particularly helpful in keeping labor pain at a manageable level. Nancy was a 25-year-old disabled woman who had had some ten or more lower-back and hip operations. As a child, she was in physical pain much of the time, pain that was particularly escalated before and after the operations. Her psychological associations with pain included being cut, being in a hospital, and being alone. During her labor she dilated to 6 centimeters and then became overwhelmed by the pain, which, incidentally, was primarily located in her lower back. She was given pain medication in such large doses that it essentially stopped her labor. After many hours, she was given Pitocin to induce labor. The Pitocin dosage caused such violent and intense contractions that she passed out with pain. She regained consciousness as she was being wheeled into the operating room for a Cesarean delivery. She awoke from the surgery in pain, in the hospital, and all alone.

During her individual sessions, she was able to release the emotional charge on these experiences and to consciously understand her previous mental associations with pain. She affirmed a new meaning of pain for several months. When she became pregnant for a second time, she opted for a VBAC. Nancy affirmed herself by saying that *labor pain* is *labor gain*. Her second child was born vaginally after eleven hours of labor pain and gain at a birth weight of almost 2 pounds greater than her first child.

Pain, then, is experienced differently and uniquely, and is based on cultural expectations, previous painful events and subsequent resolutions, and one's own present-day resources. It is possible, now, to understand our own cultural approaches to pain as described here, to release historical pain and accompanying emotion in order to achieve resolution and to increase one's own personal resources through positive thinking and realistic expectations. However, in the final analysis, each of us as women must come to respect our own inner needs, feelings, and decisions. Choosing medication during labor should not become for any woman a source of self-punishment. Women seek medication because other psychological supports and interventions have been unavailable or because they simply have gone as far as they can go without relief, or both.

Psychological Support for Fear Reduction

Studies of husband-supported childbirth indicate the psychological effects of emotional support on pain and pain tolerance (Bradley 1965). The nature of support will be discussed in a later chapter, along with the importance of communication during labor.

Pain causes fear, vulnerability, mental stress, and tension. Women need reassurance, good information, loving protection (supportive to them as mature, competent adults). They need uninterrupted contact, respect, and comfort far more often than drugs. They need positive and realistic attitudes, and creative, emotionally conscious birth teams.

It is, however, incumbent upon us to make informed choices based on accurate information. There are many reliable sources of data regarding medications, including Suzanne Arms's book *Immaculate Deception* (1975), *Right from the Start*, by Gail S. Brewer and Janice Greene (1981), *Silent Knife*, by Nancy Cohen and Lois Estner (1983), and Robert Mendelsohn's book *Mal(e)Practice* (1981).

Once drugs, their effects and risks, are understood, medication can be chosen as a last resort and with truly informed choice, free from dramatic reenactments of damsel-in-distress fairy tales in which we are robbed by ourselves and others of inner strength and confidence. Then, and only then, can women feel that they have done their best, regardless of outcome.

Preparing the Mind for Labor

In preparing for pain in labor, then, the Western woman can remain as conscious and aware as possible on the reality of labor pain. She can stay emotionally awake and intelligent on the preparation techniques presented to her. She can use her own intuitive power to evaluate those techniques by asking herself whether they support psychological notions of release and surrender, or, on the contrary, are they tension-producing, control- and discipline-oriented models.

Today's pregnant woman can take the time to assess her own beliefs and experiences of pain. She can list those beliefs about pain and ask herself whether those beliefs are conducive to positive birthing or not. When they are not supportive beliefs, she can release the emotional charge on historical events by writing the events or sharing them with a friend until a peaceful mental state is achieved. Further suggestions are contained in Chapter Eight.

Men can ask the same of themselves. The importance of a male partner's view of pain, in terms of his own realistic and informed prenatal preparation, will be further explored in Chapter Seven.

Finally, and most importantly, each of us can recognize ourselves as the unique beings that we are. We can recall our own resources and daily affirm those resources. We can remind ourselves that we are here in life to grow and to learn. And, we can recognize that our birth experiences are a very special time in life, with many opportunities for this growth and learning to take place. *Labor and childbirth are not endurance tests,* but rather opportunities to discover deeper inner resources. Pain management is not a measurement of life strength, nor is it a grading scale of personal effectiveness. If natural childbirth is approached for anything less than growth, learning, and self-love, the psychological performance pressures will only further increase physical pain. We owe no one a performance. We owe ourselves continuous self-love.

Politics

Birth is not an isolated event of psychological, physical, and spiritual expression. It is an event within a context. Today's context includes a political battlefield of egos, injustices, emotional reactions, changing policies and procedures, and drama.

As in all dramas, there are victims, rescuers, and persecutors. In order for the politics to continue, the roles change, so that some days the consumers are the victims, whereas on other days the midwives, nurses, or physicians are the victims. The goal in winning any political battle is to be perceived as the biggest victim. Again, one must lose in order to win. (This point has been discussed in Chapter Four.)

The Great Birth Battle

Childbirth educators and consumer groups are sweeping the country with outcries for reduction and elimination of medical interventions in childbirth. There are movements to support a return to midwifery, home birthing, and all natural methods. Previously Cesarean-delivered women are seeking vaginal birth even after several prior Cesareans (see *Silent Knife* [Cohen & Estner 1983]). There are movements to include the whole family in the birthing process, from the smallest children to the oldest grandparents. These are welcomed and much-needed changes.

All of these efforts have come forth in reaction to the medical view of childbirth as an abnormal condition. Women everywhere are starting to question medications, fetal monitors, episiotomies, ultrasound, and, in fact, *all* hospital procedures. We are weary of the DES, the Thalidomide, the X-rays that are visible in our bodies and our children. But the questions are causing quite a stir.

There is a battle raging between "nontraditional" childbirth educators, including midwives and a few physicians and nurses, and the "traditional," medically oriented obstetrical groups. As the former are composed primarily of women and the latter of men, this battle has become, in addition, a battle of the sexes, where the women are condemned as raving hysterics and the men as pompous know-it-alls. The battlegrounds include conference tables, physicians' offices, hospital administration meetings, and, worst of all, labor, delivery, and birthing rooms.

The battle may develop over the construction of a birthing room; a physician's unwillingness to support a VBAC due to an adherence to the outdated Craigin view, "Once a Cesarean, always a Cesarean" (Cohen & Estner 1983); or unwillingness to support a home birth or a midwife's role in childbirth. All these battles may need to be fought—if only to raise consciousness—but they are ineffective unless they are engaged in with responsibility and knowledge.

Everyone Is a "Victim"

Consumers, for example, become victims when we remain unconscious and uninformed and believe that others have a power, rather than simply a knowledge, that we do not have. Consumers also become victims when they approach medical establishments from the position of angry child, prepared to be violated rather than stand up for themselves when violations are pending.

Physicians, for example, become victims (of our anger) when they pretend to be omnipotent and misuse their knowledge to control and impose policies rather than to communicate with and understand people. Misuse of power can cause death, while proper knowledge can save lives.

Responsibility includes a willingness to understand our own participation so that we have power to change. Waiting for someone else to see the light will not make for constructive change and will only further support female scripts of powerlessness. Genuine power comes from within, not from attempting to usurp or recover it from someone else. Blaming our physicians causes damage to us both psychologically—by rendering us consistently weak—and physically—by causing us to hold anger and resentment in our bodies, to turn into ulcers, headaches, unhealed episiotomies, and unhealed Cesarean incisions.

For years, we have gone to our physicians as psychological parents and fail-proof practitioners. We have trusted in their decisions and believed that they were omnipotent because we were afraid that illness or injury might lead to death—and we wanted (naturally) to be saved.

Medical Schools' Inadequate Psychological Training

Medical school teaches doctors to unite in mutual support for policy, to ignore emotions, to work long hours without rest, and to deny personal needs for closeness, warmth, and affection. It is not training in psychological well-being, creativity, or emotional expression. We want our medicine men and women to understand our emotional needs. Yet, no one has trained them to respect, understand, or appreciate their own.

Dr. Robert Mendelsohn (1979) writes, "During eight to ten years of medical education and training, doctors are taught to believe they are God. After a few years of enormous power over life and death, they begin to believe it." "God" is not allowed to be in conflict, make a mistake, or say the wrong thing. How painful the pressure to be perfect every day! How nightmarish to live covering up mistakes because the psyche is so vulnerable that it cannot bear to admit that a "policy" or "procedure" could be incorrect!

The psychological dilemma for modern-day obstetricians is one of great conflict. We consumers demand what they have not been taught. We grant a power to cure that is greater than reality. We demand that doctors and nurses act humanly, yet criticize their smallest mistakes.

These observations are not offered to excuse harmful obstetrical practices or self-righteous medical views that are not conducive to maternal well-being. Rather, they are offered so that we might view the politics of childbirth as something we have power to change.

Medical personnel have their own responsibilities, which include a truthful look at the realities of obstetrics. Change has been painfully and dangerously slow.

The High Cost of Doctors' Pride

For more than two centuries, a mysterious disease known as childbed fever terrorized childbearing women. The mysterious fever would lead to delirium, convulsions, and death. In 1861, Ignaz Semmelweis, a Viennese physician, published a book pointing to the fact that "childbed fever" did not occur in home births or in wards run by nuns and midwives. Rather, it occurred in the wards attended by physicians (Arms 1975). The cause of this disease, Semmelweis stated, was the doctors' unwashed hands. Semmelweis was ostracized by his own colleagues, who were horrified by his assertions. In fact, in 1929, some sixty-eight years later, 40 percent of all maternal deaths were still caused by childbed fever (Arms 1975). We cannot wait seventy more years for the dangers of drugs, unnecessary Cesareans, and other risky obstetrical procedures to be corrected, nor can we correct them out of rage and powerlessness—as justified as our rage might be.

Newtonian physics states that for every action there are equal and opposite reactions. For example, the Marshes have decided to hire a well-known midwife to attend and assist at their birth. As Mrs. Marsh feels slightly fearful of home deliveries, the couple decides to birth in a community hospital. Their physician is away, and the doctor covering does not believe in the concept of labor support. He is overtly annoyed at the midwife's presence, although in reality is probably frightened, as he notices that the trio is doing well without him. The baby crowns, and the doctor steps forward. The midwife stands in front of him and directs the husband to massage the perineum so as to avoid an episiotomy. The physician jumps in front of the midwife and slips a small knife from under his sleeve and performs his routine episiotomy. A painfully true demonstration of Newtonian physics, and another violated mother.

In Hospital or at Home?

Within the politics of birthing, a current surge of debate has arisen over hospital versus home birthing. Historically, obstetrical care by male obstetricians was available to upper-class women, who could afford such services. Lower-class women were attended by midwives and family members. Today, the trend is quickly reversing, as middle- and upper-class women are seeking midwives and birth attendants at their own financial expense, while less well-off women are more likely to be attended to by the male obstetrician alone. This trend has brought to the forefront many strong opponents of hospital birthing and many courageous couples who deliver their children at home—often without the genuine support of their family, friends, and physician. Sheila Kitzinger (1981) writes, "Childbirth education is instruction to help women face the challenge of being in the alien environment of the hospital." As far back as Dick-Read, environmental influences on childbearing have been viewed as potential sources of fear. Today, our hospital birthing practices are more frightening than ever, with much new, untested (over time) equipment and more highly charged emotion caused by political quarrels inappropriately held in delivery and birthing rooms.

Informed Consumerism: Keep Your Eyes Open

Much has been written by Dr. Robert Mendelsohn in his works *Mal(e)Practice: How Doctors Manipulate Women* (1981) and *The Confessions of a Medical Heretic* (1979). Mendelsohn believes that "virtually every aspect of modern obstetrical practice conspires to isolate the mother in unfamiliar surroundings," even though studies have consistently shown that "fear is neutralized by comfortable, familiar surroundings and the support and comfort of friends" (Mendelsohn 1981). Mendelsohn says that "labor rooms have all the appeal of a prison cell," and warns women that behind the window dressing of birthing rooms lies the drugs, monitors, and attitudes that rob women of their natural ability to give birth (ibid.). His views are supported by the previously mentioned studies of Dr. Lewis Mehl (1970), which demonstrate a decrease in infant morbidity and Cesarean delivery in home birth, along with a greater sense of psychological gain.

On the other hand, medical interventions, although terribly misused, also have validity under certain conditions. Most experts on the subject of childbearing estimate that 92 to 96 percent of all births would probably go well without intervention and need not be the products of a technologically oriented medical community (see Cohen & Estner 1983; Kitzinger 1980, 1981; Marieskind 1979; Mendelsohn 1979, 1981). In rare instances, medical procedures save lives. Because of the frequency of misuse of these procedures, however, informed couples are fearful of *any* intervention and may take a reactionary rather than an informed position. As consumers, again, informed choices are more personally rewarding and psychologically fulfilling than reactionary, emotion-laden positions. It is very important that couples who believe in home birthing continue to do so, but with all options always available. It is our only hope for institutional change. As Kitzinger (1981) says, "Any system can be improved only when there are alternatives to that system." She goes on, "Hospitals are not good enough to provide an environment suited for a peak experience of one's life, not for the birth of a family."

Women who opt for hospital birthing will do well to choose their physicians carefully and their hospitals wisely, with maternal well-being as the primary goal always. Michelle Harrison, a physician who attempted a residency in obstetrics/gynecology and left because she was so appalled, recently wrote her account in *A Woman in Residence* (1982). In her dedication she writes, "To the women who entrusted me with their care at Doctors Hospital—whose forgiveness I ask for the times I did as I was ordered." Harrison could no longer go on watching women's bodies being treated as contaminated, and their integrity and control stripped away. Choosing physicians who respect women's bodies, honor women's integrity, and support women in birth, is vital. Although Harrison's descriptions are painful to read, the realities cannot be denied, nor should they be accepted.

The Ultimate Goal: Well-Being for All

With well-being as the primary goal, women are far less likely to become victims of political obstetrics, far more likely to know when they have been victimized, and more likely to be able to respond appropriately. We recommend that couples who choose hospital settings take the time to mentally clear themselves of all prior mental associations regarding hospitals, such as the broken leg, tonsillectomy, or prior birth. These experiences often promote helplessness, fear, further injury, or other emotional upset. We encourage women to walk the hospital halls singing and couples to dance at least three dances in the hospital lobby in order to disengage previous associations with hospitals that might be painful and to institute positive, joyful feelings in a place often full of disease and sorrow.

Carol's Story

The following is a letter received from a woman named Carol, describing the politics of birthing and the results. Her story may serve to remind all of us of the tragedy of mishandled emotion and uncooperative obstetrical practices. In these cases, probably the only psychological remedy for attaining genuine peace of mind is forgiveness—of ourselves, our spouses, educators, physicians, and God.

> *I had had a Cesarean delivery in 1978 with my first child. I believe now that it was not necessary in that I seemed to be progressing and I didn't feel like quitting. My doctor told me I just wasn't moving along fast enough and said he wanted to give me a little something to speed things up. He was abrupt and set up the I.V. before I could figure out what was happening. Well, to make a long, painful story short, I was given something that made my labor so violent I couldn't stand it. I begged for a Cesarean, a scene I still feel ashamed of.*
>
> *In 1981, I got pregnant again. I decided to try for a vaginal birth since a friend of mine had given birth in Europe after a Cesarean and had written to tell me I didn't necessarily need to have one. I checked it out and found that it was possible but not popular. I attended classes for VBAC mothers and planned for a hospital delivery with a midwife and my husband. When I got to the hospital [in the Boston area], I was told that I wouldn't be allowed in the birthing room because I'd had a previous Cesarean. Although the birthing room was empty and located only a few feet from the labor room, I was placed in the labor room with another couple. It was awful. I begged to be moved but didn't have the strength to labor and fight at the same time. I felt punished as I knew VBAC's weren't well received, but I didn't expect it to be this bad. I had a vaginal delivery but not without an unnecessary upset. I left the hospital almost immediately because I ruffled so many feathers I was afraid of further retaliation for my son and me. I'm angry still and hope someday to stop punitive policies.*

Power

As children in Western culture, we are well trained to respond to approval or disapproval from our parents. In "Structural Symbiotic Systems:" (1975), Dr. Robert D. Phillips describes transactional exchanges that produce adapted behaviors in their earliest forms. He refers to the simple exchange of smiles and frowns—the smile indicating mother is pleased, the frown indicating mother is displeased. The smile of approval and frown of disapproval are still emotionally activating experiences for most Western adults, especially in situations with perceived authority figures. Sondra Ray, in *Loving Relationships Training* (1980), describes parental disapproval as one of the five most important areas for resolution in order to achieve a loving relationship. Parental disapproval, as she describes it, is an invalidating experience that is a result of a legacy of disapproval and criticism that passes for protective parenting.

Women as Powerless

Female tendencies to discount inner feelings and thoughts were discussed in an earlier chapter. Colette Dowling, in *The Cinderella Complex* (1981), described this condition: "[B]ecause of a profound, deep-seated doubt in their own competence which begins in early childhood, girls become convinced that they must have protection to survive." In their research, Kagan and Moss noted that passivity and dependence toward adults appears consistently in girls and in women (Kagan, Moss & Siegel 1963). Power is perceived as being in the hands of others.

The fear of disapproval inherent in Western child-rearing practices and the female programming in self-doubt combine to create an obstetrician-patient relationship rarely perceived as having equality. Due to this inequality, our physicians play many psychological roles for us. They might be representatives of the kind, all-knowing parent we sought in childhood and keepers of knowledge about our physical health. There is probably a secret desire in most of us to remain children in some way, either to correct the hurtful events of childhood or to luxuriate once again in the protective love of a parent. We act this secret feeling out every time we seek advice rather than information. It seems to be part of our Western human condition.

"Authority" and Its Legacy of Fear

Even the best informed, psychologically prepared woman may have feelings of inferiority or helplessness in the presence of an obstetrician, nurse or other "authority." It is important to understand that the power of childbearing belongs to women. As Coleman Romalis writes in *Taking Care of the Little Woman* (1981):

Pregnancy and childbirth are uniquely feminine processes, and the latter, especially, is an area in which—it would be presumed—the woman is the dominant character. Yet, oddly enough, we find in North American society that the "expert" status has been usurped by (usually) male physicians, and it is they who have defined the roles of the various participants in the process and controlled the settings within which the process occurs.

It is equally important to understand that a few sessions in childbirth education will not defy the early childhood training that instilled fear of authority. In fact, several years of intensive psychotherapy will probably not completely erase all traces of fear and guilt over an authority's disapproving words or frown. This is not meant to take a defeatist stance in any way, but rather to understand the psychological realities inherent in most obstetrician-patient relationships. Recognizing these realities with conscious awareness can lead to well-informed choices in obstetrical practitioners and acceptance of one's own inner fears and resistance to confrontation.

Much has been written about choosing a physician wisely. Shelly Romalis, in "Natural Childbirth and the Reluctant Physician" (1981), warns against certain responses and describes several common doctor-patient exchanges that do not support female competence, such as:

(a) Woman: "I would like to have all-natural childbirth."
   Doctor: "Of course. If you think you can, I'll go along with it."
(b) Woman: "I would like to have my baby without drugs."
   Doctor: "I'm totally in favor of this, *but*, women who have set ideas in the beginning usually scream when the going gets rough."

Choose "Authority" Wisely: Stay in Charge!

Choosing a physician or midwife wisely is important not only in obtaining useful information and minimizing the inequality inherent in doctor-patient relationships, but also because of the subtle psychological power of even the most offhanded remarks made in the examining room. In the positive birthing for VBAC seminars, most women reported being told very early on in their pregnancies that their pelvises were too small, or were very small, and not adequate for vaginal delivery. With a 96 percent success rate of VBAC out of 175 or so mothers, Nancy Cohen and her clients clearly cracked the myth of the small pelvis for many women. Yet such a suggestion can be the seed for an unnecessary future Cesarean. The vulnerability to suggestion is heightened by the normal fear and apprehension of pregnant couples. One woman, Melissa, shared that she had been pregnant ten years earlier and had miscarried. At the time, she had gone for a monthly check-up on Friday and was fine. As she was leaving the office, her physician said she was in great shape, and warned her not to worry if she miscarried since one-third of all first mothers did. He said she would be in good company if she failed this time. The words ran through Melissa's head all night. The next morning she miscarried suddenly without much warning. She even consoled herself with her physician's words, until she realized what he had said. Perhaps Melissa would have miscarried in any event. It is far more useful to receive realistic, accurate information, and genuine support and encouragement, than unnecessary projections of fear and tragedy.

Peaceful Environments, Not Battlegrounds

In addition to wise choices in obstetrical care, conscious awareness of feelings of inadequacy can aid all of us in choosing our birthing environments, interventions, and attendants from a clear psychological state rather than a more emotional or childlike position. Consciousness can assist us in warding off self-recrimination brought on by our not being able to muster the strength to confront our individual physician or the system. Rather than punishing one's self with inner criticism, such situations can better be used for further consciousness raising and for strength and confidence building for future exchanges. It does not serve the primary goal of maternal well-being for women to suffer over what they should have done or said during childbirth, or to spend future years overcompensating with ongoing patient-doctor battles, battles that do not serve well-being.

The influence of the physician may be great. The power of women is increasing. Self-love and forgiveness must remain constant so that, in those genuine or perceived critical childbearing scenes, women can choose wisely and forgive themselves immediately. Jane's report can perhaps demonstrate this point.

Jane's Story

I was prepared for natural childbirth. I did not even know about Cesarean sections, but I was taking a long time and my doctor asked me if I wanted my child to be born without a head. So I agreed to a Cesarean. This was my first child and I was 28. We were married for five years before her birth and she was very wanted, as about three of those five years were spent trying to "get" Kim.

Anyway, they gave me gas. I remember I was so "sick" after that I didn't even want to see the baby, and don't remember when I did. Here transformed was a parent that had taken natural classes and had the tape recorder and camera ready.

Lastly, I had come into the hospital with one spot of poison ivy on my wrist. I told the doctor that before the "op." He said it didn't matter. They put the I.V. there and the poison ivy spread all over my arm. It was so oozy the nurses didn't want to touch it. So here I was, a first time mom: C-section with poison ivy trying to nurse a baby. Nerves—husband a perfectionist—and nervous about the situation over critical in-laws. Me—a people pleaser—Help!

I criticized myself for years, feeling that I **should** have stopped my doctor from cutting me; stopped the nurse from putting the I.V. into my poison ivy; stopped my in-laws from criticizing me; stopped my husband from harassing me. I finally realize that I should stop punishing me for doing my best in the first place.

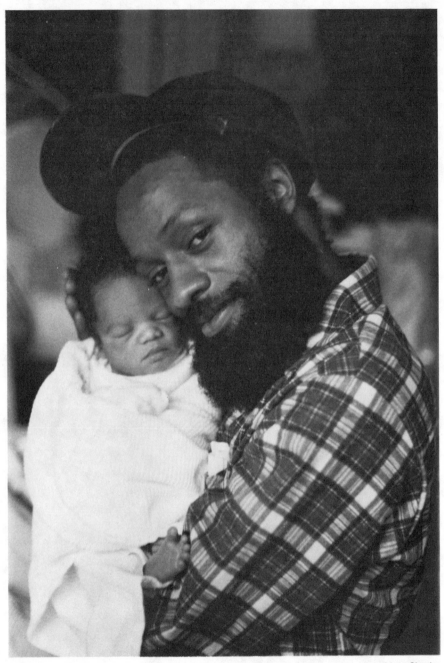

©Jean Shapiro

7

The Birth of a Father

A Father's View

John wrote this report a week after his son's birth in 1978. John's wife had a normal vaginal delivery, and the baby was a healthy 9-pounder.

This past week has been the most exciting week of my life. Things began to happen early morning on Thursday, February 2nd. My wife began having consistent contractions about seven minutes apart. We called the doctor, as first parents probably do. He said we could come in at our regularly scheduled appointment later that morning. I had a meeting so I went to work for the morning and left my wife at her mother's until about 1:00 p.m. Even that felt like abandonment.

The good news was that she was already a couple of centimeters dilated with lots of effacement. We drove home and took an afternoon nap, but constantly we were thinking about when our baby would come. We thought we'd be leaving for the hospital sometime that evening since my wife was still having steady contractions at about seven minutes apart. The contractions increased to five minutes apart and grew slightly in intensity. We stayed awake watching television until 1:00 a.m. because we were too excited to sleep. By 2:00 a.m., I fell asleep for a couple of hours. My wife dozed off between contractions. Friday morning arrived and we were still holding steady at five minute intervals. Although twenty-four hours had passed since the contractions started, we were still full of enthusiasm, energy and excitement.

We left for the hospital mostly because we were overly optimistic and needed to check progress. My wife was examined and the nurse reported that she was five centimeters—half way! We were so hopeful and delighted.

Four hours later our physician came. He reported she was only three centimeters. I thought I'd die in disappointment, after watching my wife labor for twenty-four hours to dilate one centimeter. All my dreams of natural childbirth were gone. I just couldn't imagine how we could go on. The disappointment was overpowering.

That afternoon was the longest day of my life. It was also the most alone time in my life. Contractions stopped for a while. The waters were still intact and our baby seemed lifetimes away. My wife was despondent but somehow she carried on. I felt so helpless. I wanted to trade places with her. I wanted someone to give her drugs to ease the pain or just put her under and take the baby. Then, something happened around 2:00 p.m. Contractions picked up. We stopped all the huffing and puffing we'd so regularly practiced. We stopped focusing on flowers and became completely engrossed in each contraction. Without words, we kept nurses away. Like the Eskimo custom of keeping the husband and wife together in the igloo until the child arrives, we physically closed others out and did our miracle.

My wife sank deeper and deeper into her own body. I could not communicate with her in a normal way. She asked me to repeat the phrase, "You can make it—You can make it"—almost like a mantra and in rhythm with her inner circular breathing. Our physician arrived at 6:30 p.m. and examined my wife. He announced that she was completely dilated. The waters broke and my wife began to push. The physician left and we moved into a new, active stage. My wife released these beautiful gutteral sounds. I get chills thinking about those sounds. She pushed with such determination. After forty hours of labor, no sleep and incredible strength, I saw the top of our baby's head. It disappeared and then with a push, I saw it again. I got the nurse who was shocked by the rapid progress. She (the nurse) told my wife to slow down and wait for the physician. My wife said, "Fry an egg! I'm not waiting for anybody. So get ready to catch." Three more pushes, our son was born. Our physician was upset he'd missed the delivery. We were thrilled because we felt we had done it all ourselves.

The rest of the week was the most emotionally upsetting, exciting, traumatic and lonely time of my life. I wish I'd known these things were normal. I wish they'd told us to relax and not work so hard huffing and puffing. I wish I could express all my feelings. I think I deserve to celebrate. I wish I could. Is there something wrong with me? I guess I'm just getting used to the idea that I'm a real father and I'll never be a "son" in the same way again.

A Changing Role

As recently as the 1960s, fathers were expected to wait for the "news" of their children's births away from labor and delivery rooms, alone in a hospital lobby. How often the television portrayal of birth would show the father impatiently pacing back and forth in a ten-by-six hospital waiting room. Today, it is not only expected that fathers will be involved in childbirth, but they are defined as "coaches" by such systems as the Bradley method, and they are expected to provide psychological and emotional support necessary to childbirth (Bradley 1965). There are systems that expect the father to ward off medical interventions and to be the buffer between hospital personnel who offer unwanted interventions and birthing women. Some men are psychologically prepared for participation and others are not. To truly understand the male in childbearing and the accompanying normal psychological stress, it is important to discuss the influences of male programming, of male sexuality, and of individual historical experiences activated in men during pregnancy and childbirth.

Influence of Sex-Role Scripting

It is well known, but worth repeating, that Western men are programmed in cognitive development over emotional development, and that they are taught to place great importance on maintaining control at all costs. In previous chapters, the notion of script or life drama was discussed. In the transactional analyst's view of repeated life dramas, there are common childhood messages that become inner commands for script formation. Brian Allen, in an article entitled "Liberating the Manchild" (1972), described four common male messages: "Don't lose control"; "Don't ask for help"; "Dominate women"; and, "Never be satisfied." These are hardly sound mental frameworks for positive living or positive birthing. It should also be noted that vulnerability to past injunctions and attributions increases under stress. Claude Steiner, in *Scripts People Live* (1974), describes several common male scripts that evolve out of such programming, including "Big Daddy," "Jock," "Intellectual," and "Playboy." "Big Daddy" is personified in "Marcus Welby" and "Father Knows Best." He relies on being able to rescue others in order to feel okay about himself. "Jock," represented by the "Iron Man," has devoted himself to competitive pursuits that deny emotional needs and repress acceptance of adult life. "Intellectual" believes in using his mind as a means of feeling okay and finds great difficulty in emotionally charged situations that cannot be solved by higher learning. "Playboy" searches for the perfect woman through most of his life in order to validate his sense of all-rightness, a validation often confronted when the (his) perfect-size-9 woman partner is nine months pregnant and 40 pounds heavier than his mental pictures of perfection.

Male Programming—King of the Castle?

In their work *Expectant Fathers* (1978), Sam Bittman and Sue Rosenberg Zalk interviewed a large group of fathers during both the pregnancy process and their postpartum adjustments, noting psychological upheaval in their lifestyles, marriages, sexuality, role identities, and sense of self. They found that men were eager to discuss their feelings and seemed pleased to have someone so willing to listen to them. This suggests, perhaps, that men need to create for themselves, with our support, more opportunities to release childbirth-related feelings and experiences. Bittman and Rosenberg Zalk describe the essence of male programming as calling for men to be "in control" and "on top of things" and "to wear the pants" in the family. Pregnancy and childbirth are often confrontations to such programming, when contractions are strong and the man has no power or control to ease the woman's pain. Postpartum months, when a crying baby demands great attention, are further affronts to the "king of the castle." Psychological difficulties arise not so much in the confrontation of past training, but in the expression of resulting upsets that is so severely limited by all sex-role programming. As Hogie Wycoff writes, "A particularly unhealthy result of our male-female sex-role training is that gaps have been created in people which severely limit their potential for human growth" (Steiner 1974). Conscious awareness of these limitations provides the key to freedom of expression and psychological resolution.

Men as Protectors

Men begin to know their babies indirectly through their women partners. Their energies are activated toward protecting their pregnant partners, while women are more directly concerned with protecting children. This is generally true in Western societies among nonpregnant couples as well. Most Western men, for example, would not awaken their female partners in the middle of the night to go downstairs to check on possible burglars, nor would most Western women go alone to check. This phenomenon is exacerbated in pregnancy and childbirth. Understanding the basic pecking order of protection can help to explain why men might be more concerned about their wives or female partners during labor and delivery than women, whose primary energies are dedicated to the well-being of the child. A recent review of sixty interviews with couples involved in our seminars revealed that several women felt that their husbands were not as concerned about or connected to their babies as they should have been, and that these behaviors were defined as unsupportive by the women, even though, in most cases, they felt the husbands had been very attentive to the women themselves. Once female subjects discussed the "protection system," they reported feeling less upset with their male partners and more appreciative of the latters' efforts.

"Cognitive Male" vs. "Emotional Female"

Further, it was found that many women (some 65 percent) of the sample interviewed expressed some negative feelings toward their male partners for not expressing enough emotion and for not fighting medical interventions hard enough. Western sex-role scripting permits cognitive development in men and limits emotional development with such thoughts as, "Big boys don't cry." Women, on the other hand, have more permission to be nurturing, warm, emotional, and expressive. In fact, in many relationships, the woman often expresses the emotions for both people, so that she cries for two and yells for two. For purposes of this discussion, these differences must be understood. Couples who teach themselves to bridge the cognitive-emotional gap with genuine understanding, communication, and support can far more easily adjust to the stresses of childbearing and parenting without the woman feeling "unloved" because emotion does not come forth, or the man feeling that his woman partner is hysterical and over-reactive because emotion does come forth. Gayle Peterson, in *Birthing Normally* (1981), noticed that couples with noncommunication problems and nonsupport problems can have difficulty with childbearing. Peterson says that the stress of fighting a mate causes a physical reaction that decreases uterine blood flow, leading to increased risk of fetal distress. Nancy Cohen, in her book *Silent Knife* and in her VBAC classes, teaches the simple principle that love births babies (Cohen & Estner 1983). She encourages couples to do anything they can to bring support, communication, and understanding to their relationships in order to create the optimum atmosphere for childbearing. Understanding and respecting our differences may be the first step toward the mutual respect necessary for positive birthing.

The Pregnant Father

Men experience pregnancy, childbirth, and the postpartum period physically, emotionally, and spiritually. Physically, men often report many similar symptoms to their female partners, such as nausea and weight gain. In 1965, Trethowan studied male responses to pregnancy with a group of over three hundred expectant fathers. He noticed emotional and physical symptoms in his subjects much like those of their female partners, including higher levels of anxiety than his control group, and insomnia, general restlessness, depression, and headaches. Men are often faced with fears for their own body's condition, their health, and ultimately their own mortality. They are confronted with their own sexuality, their maleness, and their feelings about the changes in their partner's body.

As a woman is reviewing her relationship with her mother, so does a man review his relationship with his father as he prepares to embrace fatherhood. He considers his father's parenting style and reevaluates his entire child-rearing.

Men are often faced with added financial responsibilities and added fears about survival, especially in these stressful economic times. And it is in this atmosphere that we have called upon men to somehow buffer their female partners from some unnecessary medical interventions during labor, a difficult task even under less stressful circumstances.

The role of fathers is changing. Hopefully, we will liberate men from superhero expectations and give them the emotional room for expressing the stresses and inadequacies we believe most men feel during this life transition. Such expression may well be the beginning of a lifetime of shared family experiences.

Support for Paternal Involvement

Most of the literature seems to indicate that husband-supported childbirth increases the mother's ability to birth naturally and with less stress. This concept became popular with the introduction of the techniques of Lamaze, where breathing in patterns was offered to improve coping capacities; of Dick-Read, who sought to increase the environmental supports for childbearing women; and of Bradley, who introduced the notion of husband as coach, providing male partners with an active and defined role. The principles of paternal participation are sound. Evidence seems to show that fathers who bond with their infants at birth have a more connected and active relationship with them in the future. In an article on father-infant attachment, Lewis Mehl (1979) stated, "[T]he father's presence at birth established nurturing patterns that continue throughout infancy and beyond." Ina May Gaskin, author of *Spiritual Midwifery* (1977) and attendant at a large number of births, wrote:

> We have noticed that there is a process of bonding between the father and child as well. Fathers who witness the birth of their children seem to form an especially close attachment to these children, and like their mates, have profound spiritual experiences as well.

It has been assumed that fathers who participated in childbirth education felt psychologically and emotionally prepared for birth. It has been assumed that the actual classes provided some arena for paternal participation that assisted men in establishing a role and identity in childbirth and that aided in overall family adjustment. However, a rather frightening (although not conclusive) study in 1976 indicated that childbirth preparation did not increase a man's sense of belongingness and failed to adequately prepare men for what was to follow birth (Wente & Crockenberg 1976). Other studies indicated a strong need on the part of men for some sense of a role within the family once the stress of childbirth and the postpartum period had thrown the family system into upheaval (Fein 1976). In our seminars, involving several hundred men to date, only one reported being asked if he wanted a drink of water during labor and none reported being physically touched by anyone other than their own female partners as a form of psychological support. These studies and experiences tend to indicate that even today's well-meaning systems for husband-supported childbirth do not adequately prepare men for the profound psychological stresses and changes normal to childbearing. As long as men are not adequately prepared, they will remain outsiders to the process, although their bodies might be physically present. Genuine involvement may help to alleviate future family stresses caused by paternal absence from home life perhaps due to lack of involvement and role definition early on.

Common Emotional Reactions

Consciousness of male-female programming has been discussed as the beginning of a sound psychological approach to childbearing. Other possible feelings may include jealousy, abandonment, and confusion, much the same feelings as those of the displaced sibling. Since male participation is relatively new, most men do not have models of male roles in childbearing beyond the famous waiting-room scenes with the pacing, anxious prospective father.

Many men are confronted with feelings and emotions they have not been trained to manage effectively, so that some men not smoking a cigar or pacing the waiting-room floor may feel awkward and out of place. Bringing fathers into the birthing process was hardly the "masculine" thing to do ten years ago. It is ironic to hear men who feel ambivalent about witnessing birth being criticized for their lack of masculine courage when at another time the same act would have produced notions of "hen-pecked" attitudes and lack of macho.

A Man's Views of the Female Body

Pregnancy and childbirth also trigger a man's most inner feelings about the workings of the female body. Western men rarely receive adequate information about women in a loving way due to our religious beliefs about sexuality, which lead to suppression of natural curiosity. In fact, most men were probably yelled at for asking what was in the Kotex box or for referring to the parts of a female body—even if only to discuss the sexuality of the house cat. This lack of information, this suppression of curiosity and infliction of embarrassment and shame, has caused men to fear women's physical beings and even to view female functioning as disgusting. It is sometimes only as adults involved in loving relationships with women's bodies that these past beliefs and fears are healed.

Adolescent males often covered their shame and lack of information with gross remarks and allusions to the menstrual cycle, menstrual discharge, or the use of sanitary napkins and tampons. The smells of the female sexual organs were talked about as distasteful, and perhaps the creation of vaginal deodorants by primarily male manufacturers attests to these beliefs. In *Boys and Sex* (1981), Wardell Pomeroy (coauthor of the Kinsey report) writes:

> The trouble begins, I think, with the failure of so many parents to talk to their children about sex in an informed and intelligent manner. Parents are always saying that children should get their sex education at home, but the Kinsey group's studies showed that only 5 percent of people interviewed got their sex education from parents.

During birth, men are asked to view the workings of the female body in a way they have never experienced before. Childbirth can activate their early fears of feminine bodies and their shame of communicating with their mothers around these events. Many of these feelings can be cleared away in advance by simply processing out the man's feelings about his mother's body, until he feels calm and good inside about his mother as a physical being. This calmness and acceptance can then be recreated in the birth scene in a way that increases male love and respect for the female physical body in childbirth.

Territoriality

As married adults, we tend to carry an internal psychological sense of territoriality and intimacy. Since childbirth involves the sexual, intimate parts of a woman's body, a man may have jealous or violated feelings as the male obstetrician examines the exposed vagina of his woman partner. Although this rather sexy scene can be "understood" as clinical in its nature, the feelings of violation may still exist, since not many Western men would expect to stand by and watch their wives intimately viewed and touched by another man under any other circumstances. Intimacy territoriality has been defined by sociologists as a basic format of tribal boundaries. Yet, Western childbearing practices violate the boundary in the name of good obstetrical practices. Childbirth is sexy. It takes a sexual act to conceive a child, sexual organs to grow and birth a child, and sexual openness to release a child. (One woman commented that she did not want to think of birth as sexy because she would be afraid to have her male physician examine her so often during labor and birth. Perhaps we could decrease the number of those painful, often unnecessary and sometimes dangerous vaginal exams if we remembered how sexy childbirth really is.) Ina May Gaskin, in *Spiritual Midwifery* (1977), says that "friendliness and intimacy" make for a sound psychological approach to childbirth. Perhaps conscious awareness of territorial violations will hasten the return of the female midwife, who presents very little competition and violation of intimacy territoriality.

Influences from the Past

Along with possible sexual feelings, jealousies, and activated childhood memories about feminine sexuality, men are also vulnerable to the same birth-related histories as women. In earlier chapters, the influence of one's own birth, family childbearing traditions, and other significant births was discussed. These same influences exist in the male psyche, often with more mystery and incorrect information attached. Since the mind tends to fill in the unknown with a barrage of negative possibilities, men are even more vulnerable to childhood myths and concerns about birthing. Although childbirth education may alleviate some of this emotional charge by providing adequate physiological information, unresolved past events may still be sources of misunderstood pain.

Bruce's Story

Individual stories have also revealed the historical influences of childbearing on the male psyche. Bruce was a good example of this phenomenon. Bruce came for counseling shortly after he and his wife became pregnant for the first time. Bruce and his wife Andrea had been planning children for several years and very much wanted this pregnancy. They were initially very excited. However, as Andrea became more noticeably pregnant, Bruce became increasingly angry with her. He could not understand his anger because he was so glad to be an expectant parent. He was further confused because he and Andrea had had such an excellent marriage in every way and considered themselves good candidates as parents.

In reviewing Bruce's history, it was discovered that sex, pregnancy, and childbirth were taboo subjects in his family and were therefore not openly discussed. Further, he recalled that when his mother was pregnant with his younger sister, she did not tell him anything about it, even though he was almost 9 years old. Bruce was informed of his mother's pregnancy by his 7-year-old friend, Joey. Bruce denied the possibility, telling Joey that his mother would have said something, and that Joey must be wrong. Several months later, when Bruce's sister was born, Joey and other friends teased Bruce for being so stupid. Bruce was angry at his mother and humiliated by his lack of information. He was unable to talk to his mom since the very subjects were taboo in the first place. Once he expressed his 9-nine-old's anger and humiliation, he was able to be with Andrea in present time and enjoy the rest of the pregnancy with excitement and support.

Current Practices

"How's the Little Woman Today?"

Many childbirth preparation courses teach men to attend obstetrical visits in order to obtain information that might not otherwise be given to women by their male obstetricians. Although it might be useful for couples to go to check-up appointments together, such practices as requiring male presence for information undermines female competence and aligns male partners with physicians against women. Coleman Romalis, in *"Taking Care of the Little Woman"* (1981), describes how male physicians commonly enlist the support of husbands in order to control birthing women. Romalis believes that such psychological alliances threaten the safety of the marriage and create much justified fear in birthing women. Ina May Gaskin (1977) reminds her midwives that even as women they must have "an impeccable" relationship with the male partner in order not to "cause any paranoia in the mother."

A Set-Up for Guilt and Failure

Such childbirth preparation courses also attempt to teach male partners how to prevent their wives from receiving unnecessary medical interventions. It is assumed that men will be able to rise above their Western child-rearing and respond with equal strength to inappropriate manifestations of authority. Our interviews with sixty sets of parents indicated that in a large majority of cases, 85 percent of the sample, men did not feel that they were able to ward off all they should have and were often left feeling that they had failed to protect their women partners during labor and delivery. Even worse, 75 percent of the women were angry (in some cases years later) at their husbands for not stopping medical interventions even in cases where they may have been lifesaving. These teachings do not take into account the overwhelming drive in all of us to avoid disapproval, as was discussed in Chapter Six. It is completely unfair and unrealistic to expect men filled with emotion to respond to authority with the sometimes necessary strength, particularly in times such as the stress during birth.

Men are trained to be "chips off the old block." They are trained to imitate their fathers and to seek approval. Advancement in the business world depends on these adaptations to male authority. Male physicians, attorneys, and law-enforcement officials all represent powerful male authority figures, symbols of fathers to be pleased, approved by, and even feared. Often, it is expected that men will be willing to confront male physicians—demanding, in a way that is counter to cultural father-son programming, that the physician account for medical interventions. Even in cases of female obstetricians, men are still faced with the fears that "talking back to mother" invites.

In any event, men can be confronted with a lifetime of inner fear and disapproval during childbirth unless this approval programming is managed, and self-acceptance and self-approval are experienced within. The reports of Jason and Michael are instructive on this point.

Jason's Story

I took the classes I was supposed to take. I felt like a little kid in school when the instructor described conception, but I knew any self-respecting middle-class man with a pregnant wife went to childbirth education. I wanted to please my wife, and I was afraid to object in any case.

We went for the full ten sessions, practiced our breathing and muscle relaxation. We got a little rainbow to hang on the wall, which we both forgot to take with us from the hospital, perhaps our only way of saying how upsetting it was to be so unprepared. Panting like a dog does not make for good birthing. But that's not what I'm really upset about.

I believed in natural childbirth. I thought women could give birth without interference. I don't know if my ideas are naive. Anyway, we went to the hospital with contractions about four minutes apart. We were real excited and thought we were doing well. My wife brought a nightgown but the nurse told her not to wear it because it would get soiled. At first I thought she was worried about spilling something on it but then I understood that she meant my wife's body stuff would "soil" it.

I was given a greenish coat to wear. It was hard not pretending to be a doctor. My voice seemed to get deeper and my know-it-all attitude came on heavy. The contractions got more intense. The labor room was ordinary with wallpaper but no big deal. We'd seen it before but we wanted it to look good so we exaggerated its appeal.

The nurse who told my wife not to wear her own nightgown was asking a lot of questions about bowel movements. It seemed strange to be so worried about the body's natural functions. I started wondering if anything was wrong and feeling scared because I felt like I didn't know enough and could be easily intimidated. Also, I got this idea that I would have to protect my wife if things got heavy. I didn't know what I was going to do.

Then, the going got tough. The contractions slowed down. People started to look concerned but no one said anything. It was weird. One minute I would have given anything to relieve my wife's pain and the next minute I would have given anything to start it up again. A couple of hours went by and then a nurse arrived with an I.V. and a pole. She said our doctor had ordered something to start labor again. I tried to find out if this was necessary or dangerous but I was told not to worry, that this stuff always worked. It was almost ten o'clock. I kept imagining they wanted us to hurry so as not to bother the doctor but I don't know.

The pain got real intense. The doctor came in and strapped a monitor on my wife. Now she seemed so stuck. I didn't know what to say—I wanted to stop them. The harder I tried, the more I felt like a little boy. I knew this wasn't natural but the nurses kept telling me that it was natural because my wife hadn't taken drugs.

My wife tried to ask questions but she couldn't ride the contractions and still ask questions. The baby came fast. The doctor cut my wife. He said he needed to get the baby out and that we'd have a better sex life if he did this. He had his knife out before we could stop him. I wanted to lash out but I couldn't. I was too overwhelmed. I lost faith in doctors and in myself. I cried in my car all the way home. I let her down. It was so sad. She never blamed me but I know she was disappointed. We don't know what else we could have done. I'm just grateful to have my wife and my son. I'm not sure what to do for future children.

Michael's Story

We'd had two miscarriages before Betsy got pregnant. We both were frightened although we didn't talk about it. Betsy was over seven months pregnant and we were two weeks into our classes when she went into labor. This was not anything like we hoped for.

Betsy and I wanted our baby. She went to her physician and he sent us to City Hospital right away. The baby was born very quickly. He seemed to almost fall out. No time for anything. He was rushed to intensive care, weighing just about two pounds. We couldn't bond or do anything but pray. Betsy was so despondent and afraid our son would die. At first I was more concerned that Betsy would die. Then, I realized she would be okay, and I started to cry. I always wanted a son. Weeks passed. He was okay.

Then, we realized we felt sad. It was hard to explain because we were so grateful. I wondered if I had somehow not helped Betsy enough with housework or if I should have stopped making love to her. It was awful to keep wondering. I needed to tell Betsy but she was lost in caring for our son. It's hard to tell other men these things. I just kept them to myself. It's a relief to tell someone now.

Labor Attendants and Psychological Support

Many writers and educators today advocate labor attendants who are present to support both men and women in the birthing of children. Nancy Cohen, especially, recommends labor attendants in these days of political upheaval in obstetrical practices (Cohen & Estner 1983). She believes that informed female labor attendants provide men with welcome relief from any expectations of battling medical interventions and free them to totally support themselves and their wives, a much more realistic and relaxed approach to birth. Labor attendants may provide a much-needed psychological as well as physiological support to women. Their efforts are best directed toward the couple's support so that birth does not become women's work with male observers.

The Conscious Father

The role of the father in childbirth is probably best described as a role in the process of development. Male presence and teamwork approaches to birth seem to provide the soundest psychological principles. There are several teamwork models that perhaps help to clarify paternal roles—a clarification that Bittman and Rosenberg Zalk, in *Expectant Fathers* (1978), describe as much desired. In three preparenting fathers' groups they studied, men tended to see themselves in two functions: "to provide moral support and comfort" and "to stay out of the way." If the latter was meant in reference to women's natural ability to give birth, then it may have some truth. Unfortunately, it referred to the territorial dictates of hospital birthing.

"The Hospital-Greens Syndrome"

Whatever role a male partner chooses to play, it can only be useful if done with consciousness and awareness. For example, hospital policy often requires a man to wear hospital greens during the labor and delivery. The effect on the man is often one of some feeling of power associated with the role of the physician that causes supportive husbands to become instant clinicians. It may have the further effect of aligning the husband or male partner with the medical establishment in a way that may be frightening or victimizing to women. Kloosterman, a Dutch obstetrician, notes that men are "disguised" in hospital garb, and that this has the effect of separating a couple during a time when unity is needed (Arms 1975).

The Marathon Handler

In some sense childbirth is much like a marathon. Once given some general guidelines, marathon runners know how to breathe, to run, and to complete their race according to their own body signals. Similarly, women know how to breathe, to birth, and to complete the delivery according to their own body signals. Marathon runners who are true champions are free to stop the fast pace, and even quit the race without loss of integrity.

Maternal well-being depends on a woman's ability to set her own pace, to birth for joy, not for achievement, and to stop whenever she determines she needs to without any loss of integrity or self-approval. There is a fine line between setting high goals and accepting disappointment when they are not achieved, and setting rigid standards of personal success that promote inner failure when not met. With this framework in mind, the marathon model is offered . . . where the joy of running each mile is of greater importance than the outcome.

The Zen Marathon

Childbirth is not an athletic event and in this sense is unlike a marathon. However, it is a physical experience requiring emotional resources and external support. It requires physiological preparation and psychological resource. It might be better described as a Zen marathon, where the focus is to become centered and one with the body, to remain on purpose and directed toward a single goal and to act from the witness or higher mind within.

Because we view marathon running as an expression of ultimate physical health, a similar attitude toward childbearing may greatly aid in the altering of present attitudes that respond to childbearing as an abnormal condition requiring medical treatment.

Lastly, marathon running requires much emotional and physical support. Yet, in the final analysis each lone runner is left to reach for her own resources and is powered by her own body's energy. So, too, the childbearing woman walks her path alone while her partner supports each step, left to face the depth of his own helplessness and inadequacy in his inability to relieve her pain.

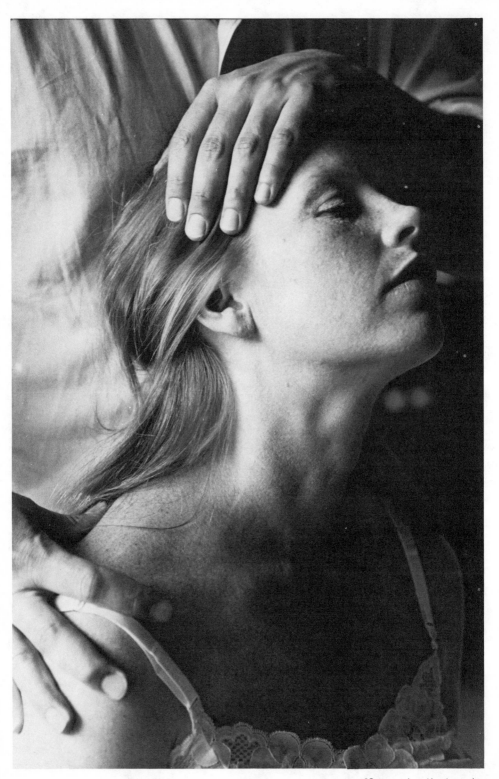

8

Positive Integration: Preparation for Birth

Many childbirth educators and psychotherapists today are using creative visualization and imagery in preparing couples for childbearing. Visualization involves mentally imagining a set of circumstances or desired outcomes so that the visualized imagery is communicated to the body. As long as their limitations and appropriate applications are understood, the principles of a physiological approach to childbirth are sound and often useful.

Along with mental imagery, various breathing techniques are also taught to childbearing couples, again with the idea that the mind can relax the body if the breathing patterns are controlled in such a way as to manage pain. Unfortunately, many breathing exercises are still being taught in the context of ego control rather than surrender. This is unfortunate, because the attitude of "control" is not conducive to body-mind integration, to pain reduction, or to total support of women's ability to birth. A further explanation and alternative systems will be offered herein. When visualization is understood and coordinated with rhythmic breathing, birth can be a highly integrated and, for many, spiritual experience.

Psychologists estimate that the mind has a mental capacity for some fifty thousand thoughts each day (Morningstar 1980). Most of these thoughts are similar in nature and tend to form clusters, often referred to as "thought patterns." These thoughts are often reflective of early childhood decisions about the nature of the world.

For example, if, when she was a child, Jane's parents were fearful of life outside the home because of lack of information about such ordinary occurrences as thunderstorms, social amenities, animals, or insects, Jane might notice herself having thoughts that express these fears. She might walk through the woods worrying about the mosquitoes, drive her car feeling fearful of a flat tire, or feel anxious about going out to dinner. In this system, the world is a contaminated, scary place, rather than a safe and loving place.

Earlier in this book, the Biblical expression of mind-body relationship was discussed. It was suggested that "what you sow in the mind, you reap in the body." Not all fifty thousand thoughts could possibly be reaped in the body. However, the primary thought patterns will be physically manifested. A common example is the person who worries a lot and develops an ulcer or a migraine headache.

Birthing and Living

Gayle Peterson (1981) based her work on the principle that as women we "birth as we live." She concluded that our beliefs about ourselves and the world will be manifested in our lives and also in our childbirth experiences. She further discovered that when women are assisted to understand their own beliefs, they may be able to alter their birthing outcomes. In our work with birthing women over the past several years, we have come to the same conclusions. The women who tend to believe that birth is frightening and dangerous are more likely to have difficult or complicated birth experiences, whether this belief was developed at their own personal birth, is a legacy of family tradition, or results from a series of frightening exchanges with birthing women as adults. For example, women who work in intensive-care nurseries or high-risk hospitals are more likely to develop a high-risk mindset that will be manifested in a complicated birth.

Emotionally Charged Beliefs Yield Outcomes

Understanding this relationship between mind and body is a significant first step toward creating a positive outcome. Understanding that, although it may be possible to examine some of our beliefs about birth, it will never be possible to reach them all, is a significant step toward a positive birthing experience. The beliefs that carry an emotional charge are the ones that we are more likely to manifest in present-day outcomes. Lewis Mehl (1979) writes, "Many women now believe in the power of technology, including women who want to deliver outside of the hospital . . . . These beliefs have become, to a large extent, internalized and emotionally charged." Such emotionally charged beliefs are not easy to relinquish, even simple ones, unless there is an opportunity for the systematic and conscious examination of those beliefs or a crisis situation that demands a creative new response. The systematic and conscious basic thought patterns unique to each individual system can be identified through the use of something such as the following "birth inventory." In completing the inventory, it should not be assumed that every negative thought produces a negative outcome. In fact, most childbearing men and women carry frightening thoughts about deformed children or complicated births. These usually pass like clouds on a windy day and are replaced by hope and confidence.

Fill out the Birth Inventory by responding to each question as spontaneously as possible. Try not to mentally strain for an answer but rather to simply fill in each question with the first ideas that come to mind.

Now that you have completed the questions, read over each answer, asking yourself this question: "Are my beliefs conducive to normal positive birthing?" Check those that are not.

Let Go of Emotional Charge

This consciousness-awareness inventory was developed out of several years of counseling and teaching childbearing women. It may assist in identifying potential trouble areas that may be the nesting ground of emotionally charged negative beliefs. Once beliefs are identified, it is sometimes possible to choose whether to act on those beliefs or not. Occasionally, the emotional charge must be released, a task that is not easily discussed within the confines of this material. As shown previously, letters used as a release exercise often allow an emotional discharge. Verbal sharing with supportive family and friends or membership in a support group can facilitate release. Some women "dream out" their feelings, others "yell or cry out" their feelings, and others can meditate their upsets away. Whatever your style, releasing emotionally charged psychic pain can greatly aid in muscle relaxation in childbearing.

Now take a minute to examine your belief systems. Rewrite all nonsupportive statements in the positive and use these new ideas and affirmations to build a new belief system.

The work of Gayle Peterson, discussed in *Birthing Normally* (1981), contains many examples of women who released birth-related upsets and went on to have relaxed, normal childbirths. She writes particularly about women who experienced some unresolved birth-related loss, such as a woman with a history of abortions and a woman who gave birth to a son and surrendered him for adoption.

Several women attending our seminars have shared that they felt afraid "to let go" of their babies as a result of a family story about someone "almost dying" in childbirth, leading to beliefs that birth is dangerous or even tragic.

If You Thought It Up—Think It Down

Dr. Joseph Murphy, in *The Power of the Subconscious Mind* (1963), writes, "The mind is the source of infinite wisdom, infinite power and an

BIRTH INVENTORY

Instructions: Answer each question as truthfully as you can. You need not be concerned about accuracy.

a. What do you believe about your own personal birth (not your child's)? (3 items)
   1. I believe
   2. I believe
   3. I believe

b. What does your mother believe about your birth?
   1. She believes
   2. She believes
   3. She believes

c. What does your father believe about your birth?
   1. He believes
   2. He believes
   3. He believes

d. What do you believe about women?
   1. I believe
   2. I believe
   3. I believe

e. What does your mother believe about women?
   1. She believes
   2. She believes
   3. She believes

f. What does your father believe about women?
   1. He believes
   2. He believes
   3. He believes

g. How would a group of women from your family (aunts, sisters, grandmothers, etc.) fill in this statement? The women in our family are:
   1.
   2.
   3.

h. How would a group of women from your family (aunts, sisters, grandmothers, etc.) fill in this statement? Childbirth is:
   1.
   2.
   3.

i. What did you believe about sex at the age of 16?
   1.
   2.
   3.

j. What does your mother believe about sex?
   1.
   2.
   3.

k. What does your father believe about sex?
   1.
   2.
   3.

l. What do you believe about pregnancy?
   1.
   2.
   3.

m. What does your mother believe about pregnancy?
   1.
   2.
   3.

n. What does your father believe about pregnancy?
   1.
   2.
   3.

o. How do you feel talking to a physician?
   1.
   2.
   3.

p. What have your friends told you about pregnancy?
   1.
   2.
   3.

q. What have your friends told you about childbirth?
   1.
   2.
   3.

r. What three words do you associate with "pain"?
   1.
   2.
   3.

s. What three words do you associate with "hospital"?
   1.
   2.
   3.

t. What do you believe about your siblings' births (if relevant)?

   1.

   2.

   3.

u. What does your mother believe about your siblings' births (if relevant)?

   1.

   2.

   3.

v. What does your father believe about your siblings' births (if relevant)?

   1.

   2.

   3.

w. What did/does your religion teach you about birth?

   1.

   2.

   3.

x. What did/does your religion teach you about sex?

   1.

   2.

   3.

y. What are your three most secret thoughts about childbirth?

   1.

   2.

   3.

z. What do you fear the most?

   1.

   2.

   3.

infinite supply of all that is necessary, which is waiting for development and expression." He believes strongly in the use of positive thought to achieve results. Sondra Ray, in her books *Loving Relationships* (1980) and *I Deserve Love* (1976), also writes of the power of the mind and suggests the use of affirmations (repeated positive thoughts designed to yield a certain outcome). Affirmations are mental suggestions intended to lead to positive results. For example, a review of the birth-belief inventory may reveal that there are a cluster of negative beliefs about sex, including such ideas as that sex is dirty, forbidden, bad, taboo, etc. An appropriate affirmation might be: "I love and respect all of my sexual parts"; "I open my sexual body and birth freely." Sondra Ray reminds us that affirmations can be done in many different ways. They can be written, thought about, spoken, or recorded and played back. Some good ideas might be: "I, Susan, deserve a totally supportive birth experience"; "I, Denise, am a competent human being and my competence is reflected in my labor and childbirth"; "I, Ann, give birth to children who reflect my highest thoughts of myself."

It is important to emphasize that affirmations work best when they are simple and easily remembered, and are repeated often. It is also important to note that affirmations create a positive mindset that may or may not take hold according to what emotionally charged beliefs remain in storage. Since it is never useful for any "soul searcher" to attempt to know every possible negative thought, use of the inventory—along with an emotional release exercise and ongoing affirmations—is adequate. The inventory is a tool for improvement and should never be used for self-punishment, especially when desired results are not consistent with actual outcomes. As my dearest friend so often reminds me: "We go as far as we can go and leave the rest to God!"

Visualization

In recent years, the use of mental control for physical healing became widely publicized by Stephanie Simonton and Carl Simonton (1978) in their treatment of cancer patients. They advocate the use of positive thinking and visualization designed to reorder disease-producing belief systems and to activate physical systems for healing and health maintenance. A major determining factor in the success of such treatment lies in the patient's emotional commitment to getting well.

The biofeedback approach to disease also borders on this approach, allowing patients to become highly conscious of physiological systems and reactions, and of reordering mind structures to reduce pain and eliminate disease. All of these techniques point to the natural tendency toward health and the body's efficient approach to healing. There are times when illness or accident may enter our lives, but even these events often occur when we most need a rest or vacation.

Childbearing is an expression of the masterpiece of the human female body. It is miraculous and mysterious, and deserves our finest attention. In order to use visualization effectively, an adequate understanding of the physiology of childbirth is essential. The earliest pioneers of childbirth preparation knew well the need for informed consumerism and also understood the relationship between fear and the "unknown." Lamaze and Dick-Read learned that by educating couples in the physiology of childbirth and pain, fear of the unknown would decrease, while relaxation would increase. Regardless of what system, if any, one chooses for childbearing, knowledge of the body is essential

The body's function during labor and delivery has been well documented by Sheila Kitzinger in *The Experience of Childbirth* (1981), Ina May Gaskin in *Spiritual Midwifery* (1977), and Gail Brewer and Janice Greene in *Right from the Start* (1981). The dangers and risks of drugs, fetal monitors, ultrasound, and other medical interventions have also been well documented in Nancy Cohen and Lois Estner's book, *Silent Knife: Cesarean Prevention and Vaginal Birth after Cesarean* (1983), and in Dr. Robert Mendelsohn's *Mal(e) Practice: How Doctors Manipulate Women* (1981), as well as in several others. Since so much well-written material is available on this subject, it will not be discussed in this work.

Ten Useful Principles for Effective Visualizations

Once the physiology of childbearing is learned and appreciated, visualization can be used to integrate and harmonize the mind-body relationship. Like affirmations, visualization is most effective when past negative belief systems become conscious and historical emotional upset has been released, as then the mental pathways are clear for new ideas, experiences, and images.

In recent years, through the work of Milton Erickson, who studied the use of hypnosis and the nature of the mind, much has been revealed about the nature of the human mind that can be applied to the art and science of visualizations for childbearing. (Rossi & Erickson 1974). Ten basic principles for effective visualizations are contained herein, along with excerpts from sample visualization exercises now in use, based on the techniques of indirect self-hypnosis. These ten guidelines can be used in creating a personal visualization tape for one's own personal use or for that of a friend or student. Instructors may find these guidelines useful in designing a general visualization process that can be practiced during prenatal class sessions.

1. RELAXATION

The mind contains a constant flow of mental chatter. Although most Western studies and observations of Eastern practitioners of meditation indicate greater health in the more relaxed brain-wave frequencies of *alpha* and *theta*, most Westerners spend the greatest quantity of time in *beta* and *delta* (*beta* being the mental chattering and *delta* a sound sleep). Therefore, visualizations are more easily accepted after some time and some suggestions to relax. Starting with closed eyes, gradually suggest to yourself or another a state of relaxation, with focus on the breath or on surrender into the chair. Abrupt commands such as "Close your eyes and completely relax" are difficult to effectuate.

Relaxation is also enhanced when the physical seating position does not require the body to support itself. Lying down or sitting up with uncrossed arms and legs is conducive to relaxing. Occasionally, it is useful to suggest relaxation, calm, peace in the body, as reflected in the breath.

2. CLEAR MIND

With fifty thousand thoughts per day, an absolutely clear mind is not possible. However, suggestions to simply observe thoughts or to allow them to pass like clouds on a windy day slow the mental chatter. Allowing subjects time to notice their thoughts and to translate thoughts into positive suggestions, such as, "You may notice the sounds of traffic going by—perhaps a reminder of how good it is to be inside where it is calm and restful," also slows down the stream of consciousness.

3. USE OF SUGGESTION

Visualization is an indirect relaxation and integration technique. Using suggestions rather than direct confrontations is more conducive to conjuring appropriate images without encountering resistance—for example, "relaxing a little more with each breath," rather than, "You are now completely relaxed." Commands produce resistance, so statements such as, "Do this," rather than, "I'd like you to imagine" may prove confrontive and may activate mental reluctance.

4. GENTLE VOICE

There are courses that teach voice control and intonation for those who are seeking highly technical data. These courses are sponsored by institutions that offer neurolinguistic programming skills (Bandler & Grinder 1975, 1976). Basically, allowing the voice to flow with the atmosphere and to guide itself can eliminate artificial adaptive qualities that distract subjects from flowing with the leader's suggestions. Placing emphasis on special words such as: Allow air to be gently taken into the body and to exhale *down* through the legs—*down* to the earth.

5. ALLOW FOR CREATIVITY

When the body and mind are opened and integrated, they serve as natural healing agents. The integration allows the body to communicate its needs to the mind. Each subject experiences a visualization according to his or her own unique system. Inviting subjects to "choose a place anywhere in the real or imagined world that offers safety and support" allows subjects to create a sanctuary that is custom designed, and is preferable to dictating that everyone "visit a beach."

6. GROUNDING THE VISUALIZATION

"Grounding" is a term that is usually applied to electrical systems and means that the wiring is rooted safely in some shockproof location point.

Grounding the mental circuitry in a safe place in order to experience the flow of energy release that may accompany a visualization is used to provide psychic safety for the subject. Breath—i.e., focusing on and listening to one's own breathing—can be such a grounding point, a grounding point that can be returned to for calmness at various moments throughout a visualization.

7. SETTING GOALS

Although we recognize the need for clear intention and goal setting, the principles of visualization prohibit direct commands and externally set goals. Telling a subject, "You are now having the ideal home birth you desire," is not as usual as suggesting that she set her own goals, guided by her own body and supported by ideals of positive birthing.

Suggesting a flow of positive images and feelings and a willingness to embrace every event of childbirth allows women to build self-confidence and competence. The mind and body already know what positive, healthy experiences are and can easily connect these energies to birth, if correctly supported. The use of such expressions as "breathing easily," "letting go," "healthy sensations," can produce images that reflect a positive feeling of a good birth experience rather than perfectionistic pictures that would be difficult to match in reality.

8. POSITIVE CONCLUSION

Visualization processes may allow subjects to relieve some difficult experience but must lead the subject to the healing and resolution of this experience. The visualizer should conclude feeling generally relaxed and peaceful, with no new or additional stresses in the body. If some stress is incurred, attention should be paid to reexperiencing a guided fantasy to unblock this stress. Otherwise, the subject may conclude that the process was ineffective and may feel angry (consciously or unconsciously) with the presenter.

9. REPETITION FOR SUCCESS

Repeated thoughts have the greatest impact. Since visualizations are guided thoughts, their effectiveness lies in the repeated, positive mental suggestion. Tape-recorded, guided fantasies can be replayed throughout the pregnancy, altering negative belief systems and producing positive, involved attitudes toward birth and the physiological process.

10. VISUALIZATION AS SELF-HYPNOSIS

All suggested mental imagery is self-hypnosis in that one is always free to accept or reject a suggestion. Due to our strong beliefs in the body's natural tendency toward health and the mind's innate desire for peace, it is further concluded that subjects naturally filter out material that is not useful, and that, conversely, they absorb everything that is supportive of health. Consumers are free to become both the presenter and the subject by recording a custom-designed visualization onto a tape (perhaps playing a favorite musical piece in the background). Whether you are the subject, presenter, or both, visualization is an exercise in enlisting all available positive resources for the purpose of a positive childbirth experience.

A Sample Visualization

The following visualization was designed by the author for the purpose of (a) creating an inner sanctuary of psychic resources for birthing; (b) enlisting support; and (c) focusing on positive outcomes.

Find a comfortable position in the room. You could be lying down on the floor, sitting against the wall, or up in a chair. Your body should be supported in a way that requires no effort on your part. Good.

Now, begin to let go of holding the weight of the body and gently give in to your chair or floor. Take a breath. Good. Now, again. Good. Just listen for a moment to the sounds of the breath. The inhale can be used to take in new and cleansing energy. Gravity is kind and will take the exhale without our effort—and with the exhale, all that is unnecessary is released and disappears.

So, breathe a few deeper breaths, allowing a slightly more relaxed feeling with each breath. Perhaps, you will feel like closing your eyes and allowing yourself to drift from this room a bit, noticing the sounds of [list whatever you hear] the heat being pumped into the room—reminding us, perhaps, of how good it is to be warm and safe inside. And then, off in the distance, the sounds of cars passing by as others go about their day. It's good to be able to slow down at times during the day, to relax the mind and the body.

Now, take another deep, cleansing breath and on the exhale gently let any thoughts you might be having pass like clouds on a windy day. Good. Now, begin to allow yourself to drift off to a comfortable, safe place that pleases you and supports you. Perhaps you'll visit a sandy beach or a rich green forest, or, perhaps, a special room or backyard that feels just right.

Once you arrive, allow yourself to breathe slowly, deeply, taking in the sights and sounds and peace of this place. Allow pleasant memories of this place, should there be some. It's good to be reminded of the peace, of the calm that we deserve, and to notice your own capacity to create these sensations at any time.

Breathe and relax into your surroundings. Now, without thinking or reasoning, look around and feel with your heart if this atmosphere would be one in which you could choose to birth a child. And just check the environment—not for its technical capacities, but rather for its sensory

*capacities—knowing that the newborn is so open to the sensory aware-
nesses, to soothing sounds, to gentle smells, and clear, clean air. And as
you look with your heart to determine the energies around you, make sure
these are the best energies you can create, since you and your baby deserve
only the best. If any alterations must be made, simply do so without effort—
by simply directing from the heart all that is good.*

*Breathe and let go—releasing into gravity. Take a moment to affirm your
ability to create now inside of yourself an ideal and sacred place within
your heart for a child to be born—a place where guilt and inadequacy are
unknown and support is abundant.*

*Good. Breathe, and as you experience peace within, bring to you now
anyone in your life—a husband, a friend, a mother, father, sister, a midwife, or any support person whose nourishing goodness you could receive
unconditionally and whose energy would honor this place with the reverence and respect you deserve. Because you are the master of this place,
you determine who will be allowed here as well as what each supporter
will bring. You can leave all unresolved conflict outside and far away from
this birth place and allow supporters to carry in their own hearts the
reverence and respect you deserve.*

*Good. Now breathe, and again examine (not with criticism, but with
compassion) each support person. Determine with a loving heart if these
are energies that you want your child born into.*

*If any energy registers anything less than the best for you and your
child, alter the energy until it provides the support your child deserves.
Good, and breathe. Now, once you have created support in its highest
form, affirm yourself for your capacity to do so. Affirm again your capacity
to create in your heart a peaceful and sacred place, and to surround
yourself with the total support you deserve. As you affirm yourself, allow
yourself to imagine the time of birth drawing near. In its magnificent
wisdom the body begins the process of labor. It knows well its inner clock.
It knows well its own rhythm. Allow all the time you need to pass between
each surge of energy—reminding yourself at every break of the natural
health of these body sensations. When enough time has passed in your
mind, whether hours or days, allow your baby to come forth into the world,
surrendering to the wisdom of the body. Take your time, since the transition
from pregnancy to motherhood demands grace and self-love.*

*Make this transition with the emotional ease of stepping over a well-
constructed footbridge—one in which each stone has been carefully placed
so that all is balanced, all is strong, capable of holding any weight.*

*And as you gracefully move in your heart from pregnancy to motherhood,
you are able to surrender to releasing your baby in a protected, supported
way, knowing that you have created in advance the place, the atmosphere,
that best supports all the sensory perceptions of a newborn.*

*As this place is a reflection of union and harmony, so now are these
moments with your child. As you are gently embraced by motherhood, so
you gently embrace your child. You and your child are surrounded by
loving and supportive energies and you are pleased with yourself for the
experience.*

Breathe, and affirm your capacity to embrace motherhood within your-self and to embrace your child. All of the events are within your capacity to create in your own heart, regardless of the external events in the world. It's good to know you have this ability for self-love, in good times and in difficult times. We always deserve a positive feeling about ourselves, no matter what the conditions. Take a moment to remind yourself of your body's wisdom to know exactly when to begin the process of labor on the physical plane. Keep with you now the connection to your baby as a source of comfort and strength to both of you.

In a few moments, you will be drifting back into the room, once again conscious of the heater or traffic or the people on either side of you. Before you drift fully back, take a moment to place in your mind a kind and loving voice—a voice that reminds you of your competence as a woman, your capacity for positive birthing, and your eternal right to self-love. This voice can be called upon at any time to speak to your heart—to remind you of these things.

Slowly, gently, come back into the room, allowing the loving voice to remain in a quiet place, waiting for you to call her. Slowly, gently, come back into the room. Begin to feel the floor or walls or chairs around you—breathing peaceful, restful sighs of relief. When you are ready, open your eyes, so I'll know you are back.

There are many variations in style and purpose for birthing visualizations. Gayle Peterson, in *Birthing Normally* (1981), describes visualization for use in relaxation of the body, as well as an actual birth visualization, including focusing on the sensations of labor and delivery as well as a view of the inner uterine world from the baby's point of observation.

Nancy Cohen, in her seminars and in the book *Silent Knife*, presents a lengthy and beautiful guided imagery to assist previously Cesarean-delivered women in the mental preparation supportive of successful VBAC (Cohen & Estner 1983). She guides women (and men) through labor, reframing pain beliefs, and building confidence in women's abilities to birth vaginally.

All childbearing women deserve the opportunity to imagine and visualize the very best for themselves.

Breathing

For centuries, breathing has been studied as a vital life force beyond the physical function of gas exchange. It has been called the *"prana"* or life force and has been the focal point of yoga practices and meditative techniques through the ages. It is only fitting that the *prana* become the integrating force between mind and body during childbirth.

Unfortunately, many present-day breathing techniques are based on incorrect psychological as well as physiological principles. Any technique that fosters discipline and control does not support relaxation and the surrender necessary for positive birthing. Ina May Gaskin (1977) says that breathing should be deep and slow. She stresses the importance of flowing with the intense body energies normal in birthing. She cautions, "The practice of panting in the first stage tends to slow the labor and can cause hyperventilation in the mother, resulting in carbon dioxide depletion." Ina May Gaskin, along with her farm midwives, has assisted at hundreds of births, with a record of 984 undrugged births out of 1,000 in the years from 1970 to 1979.

Surrendering to the Body

Techniques that encourage women to focus on meaningless objects outside their physiological process fail to support the whole concept of surrendering to the body. Distracting one's attention away from the action of the uterus negates the beauty of the birthing process and causes an incorrect flow of physical energies. In this book *Bioenergetics* (1975), Alexander Lowen wrote of the importance of aligning the body and the breath with the natural forces of gravity. Breathing up into the air away from the body causes disharmony in the physical body and further increases pain. Sheila Kitzinger (1981) warns, "If a woman tries to resist uterine contractions, or merely endure them, she will have severe pain." She continues, "Lamaze and Vellay in France taught that learning about breathing and being able to control it can help a woman by allowing her to get enough oxygen either in pregnancy or labor."

Lamaze techniques were offered at a time when no other techniques were available to birthing women. It was natural for all to accept the techniques as valuable without recognizing that the principles of informed consumerism and ability to regain some control over childbirth were the real gains for women and men. There are many women who delivered their children naturally who swear by the panting, huffing, puffing, and blowing of Lamaze breathing. It is sad to see so many women credit a technique rather than themselves and their own inner resources for their birthing experiences. Women who birth joyfully do so because of who they are, what they believe, and how they live.

Breathing for Release

Breathing for release and integration is far more useful and conducive to positive birthing. Sheila Kitzinger suggests a model for breathing in an easy, rhythmic, and relaxed way. She discusses her approach in *The Experience of Childbirth* (1981). The idea of body-mind integration through breathing is advocated by those who practice kriya yoga, an old and much-used breathing technique that views the breath as circular in motion and constant in flow. This yoga practice was the basis of Leonard Orr's rebirthing techniques as discussed in his work *Rebirthing in the New Age* (1977). Although he makes a rather drastic assumption that everyone experiences birth trauma, his techniques have been used for alternative breathing approaches in childbearing. Orr teaches students to focus on the breath and to visualize each breath as a complete circle with no beginning and no ending. Subjects report a deep sense of inner relaxation and spiritual consciousness associated with regular practice of rebirthing that has led to reports of a newfound sense of body mastery.

Breathing Is Loving the Baby

This discussion on breathing is presented for two reasons: first, to discourage the use of disciplines and false senses of control; and second, to inform consumers of the need for integrated breathing practices that support women's competence, physical process, and overall body-mind integration. The following story describes a woman's integration of breathing and mental imagery, a process she stumbled upon in her desperation to birth naturally.

> *Before Jeremy was born, we did all the "right" things to prepare for natural childbirth. We read books, attended classes and everything. I went into labor just after my due date and was thrilled to be so timely.*
>
> *I labored for almost thirty hours in lots of pain and discovered I was only 3 centimeters dilated. I was panting, puffing, and blowing my way into exhaustion. I was determined to go on but felt like I was losing my confidence quickly. I somehow allowed myself to stop all the work of breathing and conserve energy.*
>
> *I imagined my cervix like a flower opening and I breathed into the center with each contraction. After thirty hours of labor my blood pressure returned to normal and my body dilated to 6 centimeters.*
>
> *I regained faith in myself, even though I was physically exhausted. The contractions got very fast, intense and long. Imagining their productivity and their ability to open my body gave me strength to go on. I don't feel like "thanking Dr. Lamaze." My son was born after forty hours of labor and I thank "myself"!*

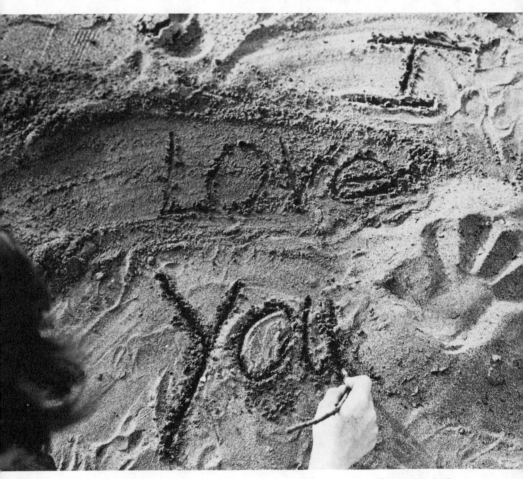

©Jackie Murphy-Knapp

9

Relationship Revival: A Pre-Birth Mini-Course

When someone says, "I love you" and means it, it opens up his throat—it literally does. And when the throat opens up, so does the cervix. I've been checking a lady's dilation at the same time she'd say that, and I could feel a distinct difference in her tissue, in how stretchy it was, that was exactly synchronous with her saying, "I love you." (Gaskin 1977)

Pregnancy is an opportunity for couples to prepare their relationship for the stresses of birthing and the challenges of parenting. Each couple brings to their birth a unique combination of energies, feelings, and thoughts that results in their relationship. Although this "relationship revival" will include much more than love, it is built on the work of Ina May Gaskin and others who so clearly understand the connection between a healthy, loving relationship and a positive birthing. Love, communication, support, and touch are four important areas for revitalization.

Love

Love, for most Westerners, is a shallow experience built on agreement rather than support, on self-righteousness and false pride rather than acceptance, and on mental pictures of "happily ever after" rather than the day-to-day realities of having a relationship. Most of us operate out of a scarcity and deficiency of love that leaves us desperate in our approach to relationships. As Ken Keyes writes in *A Conscious Person's Guide to Relationships* (1979), "We are on the lookout for people who seem to be able to accept and love us. We are like hungry tigers who haven't eaten for a month." Two desperate, hungry tigers could hardly be expected to welcome another hungry mouth to feed. So, the first step in the relationship revival is love and plenty. Love is often thought of as an emotion, a pleasant emotion that brings about enjoyable (maybe some sexy) body sensations and good feelings. Love is also connected with romantic pictures of candlelight dinners, wine, and, of course, roses. We may think it a pleasure to be one of the company of two typical lovebirds. However, if our notions of love are limited to fairy tales and old movies, what then do we bring to our childbirths? The emotions are sometimes pleasant and sometimes painful. The body sensations range from absolute bliss to excruciating pain. The candlelight, wine, and roses may take a permanent back seat to the nightlight, breastfeeding, and overgrown front lawn that has not been mowed because neither parent has the energy any more to push the lawn mower. Where is love?

It has already been established that pregnancy and childbirth are emotionally activating events and that any such stressful, emotionally charged experience activates past feelings and thoughts, including our experiences of marriage and family. It offers, then, the opportunity for personal growth as individuals and as a couple. Couples are given the chance to expand their former notions of love to include an all-encompassing state of consciousness rather than a limited mental picture or emotion. Gerald Jampolsky, in *Love Is Letting Go of Fear* (1979), writes, "Love is the total absence of fear. Love asks no questions. Its natural state is one of extension and expansion, not comparison and measurement. Love, then, is really everything of value."

No Scarcity

Plenty is exactly the opposite of scarcity ("scare-city"). In America, we have become accustomed to oil shortages that produce long lines and hot tempers at gas stations. We have seen the empty supermarket shelves that were once filled with peanut butter, while some household cabinets held thirty jars of hoarded peanut butter. We have also experienced the emotional desperation and hoarding of love innate in our system. It causes us to be fearful to give, and fearful to ask for what we need lest someone else should do without. Scarcity is indeed "scare city." Fear produces tension. Dick-Read (1944) described this condition in childbirth as the "fear-tension-pain" response. Relationships built on scarcity produce fear. There is not now nor has there ever been a shortage of love. Understanding the truth of abundance opens us up to giving and sharing, a must for relaxed, supported child-bearing.

Communication

Bradley and his followers formulated a husband-coached approach to child-birth. They recognized that laboring women seemed to have a less stressful time when supported by someone they loved and trusted. Men were and are given in this method the defined role of coach and participate actively in the childbirth process. The idea that a couple unite to birth their own child is a basically sound approach to positive family beginnings. In order to successfully team up for childbirth, a couple must have good communication skills.

Honor Your Needs

Most of us educated Westerners would probably consider ourselves well able to relate our needs, wants, and feelings. Under ordinary life circumstances, this may be somewhat true. However, under the stress of labor and delivery, communication becomes a true challenge. Labor requires an absence of dramatization and an on-purpose attitude.

It is not uncommon, for example, for birthing women to be discounted in communications. A "discount" is a term from transactional analysis that means "a lack of attention or negative attention that emotionally hurts" (James & Jongeward 1973). Because of the politics that often align men with physicians in order to control women, women are not always given accurate information. Men also fear telling their spouses the truth if some potential difficulty arises. Actually, the woman's intuition has probably already signaled "difficulty" and her imagination has supplied her with the worst possible outcome. Lack of information produces further anxiety, which only leads to fear, tension, and pain. Miscommunications cause emotional stress and can lead to physiologic distress. The following incidents of miscommunication have been reported by seminar participants.

> We arrived at the hospital and I was 7 or 8 centimeters dilated. I was really excited. My husband left me for a few minutes to check something at the admissions office. While he was gone, I became really scared, I felt alone, and I was afraid he wouldn't find me. I asked a nurse where he was and she said, "Don't worry, you're fine," but she didn't tell me where he was. My contractions got very intense. I guess I was uptight. My husband came back and I was really hurting. I asked him where he'd been and he said not to talk. I guess he wanted me to concentrate on my breathing.
>
> I started to think that something was wrong and that people weren't

*telling me. I went on with my labor. Then, I asked my husband where our doctor was and he said, "He'll be by soon." I really needed to know **where*** he was because I was still afraid that something was wrong. My labor slowed down over the next couple of hours. At the time I was glad and I wasn't conscious of my fear. Then, my labor attendant asked me what I was afraid of. I explained what had happened. My husband told me that he had been at the admissions office and that our physician was in the hospital with an emergency and would come to us as soon as he finished.

My labor started again and our daughter, Ava, was born in a couple of hours.

Cecelia and Joe were tense throughout the pregnancy. Joe had been working long hours in a new job while Cecelia had been working part time. At times, they felt worlds apart. In some ways, they were glad to be pregnant. Cecelia hoped it would bring them closer, even though she vaguely knew better. She felt unsupported in that Joe had missed a couple of childbirth classes because of work. As the birth drew near, Cecelia became more desperate to communicate with Joe.

During labor, they felt connected and were pleased that they could work so well as a team. At the hospital, Joe got hungry and took out some fruit they had packed for him to snack on. He peeled a banana. Cecelia was furious. She said that the banana was sickening, that Joe had been insensitive throughout the pregnancy and that it was his "banana" that had gotten her into this mess. He tried to defend himself with excuses about work. Their labor attendant stepped in and brought them back to their delivery, but so much energy had been lost that Cecelia asked for medication. In this situation, she might not have needed medical intervention if some of the discounted emotion had been expressed and received early on.

Purposeful Communication—The Critical Energy Contact

Purposeful communication begins with eye contact. Eye contact sets the stage for intentional exchanges. Purposeful communication means that the listener abandons all his or her mental rehearsals and predisposed ideas about what he or she will say next. As Stewart Emery writes in *Actualizations: You Don't Have to Rehearse to Be Yourself* (1978):

> When we do talk, most of us have our attention focused inside of our heads instead of where it should be, outside of ourselves. The only way we can possibly know whether we are being heard or not is to look at the people we want to be heard by and to notice whether they are hearing us.

When a couple is out of practice or has begun to take communication skills for granted, practice sessions greatly aid in reestablishing connections. Over the past fifteen years, communications workshops have been developed throughout the country by people like Sondra Ray, who designed "loving relationships training," and Stewart Emery, who designed "actualizations." The following basic communications exercise is often recommended to our pregnant and postpartum couples.

A Practice Exercise

Choose a time when you are not exhausted and have some emotional energy to devote to the exercise (perhaps early morning, after supper, or before bedtime). Choose a place where you both can sit comfortably in quiet, without outside disturbances and distractions. Sit across from each other so that you are at eye level with your knees touching, if possible. Close your eyes and breathe gently and slowly, allowing the business of the mind to become calm and peaceful (three to four minutes). Open your eyes and gaze into each other's eyes without any words. Remember that this is not a staring contest and that nonverbal intimacy outside of sex can be an unfamiliar or even uncomfortable experience. Allow any feelings that are there to simply be there. If you feel like laughing or crying or yawning, feel free to do so. Stay in the exercise for at least five minutes before closing your eyes.

Again, close your eyes and breathe slowly and deeply, allowing the exhale to release any stress or tension. Take one minute or so to relax.

Then, open your eyes and decide who will share first. Assume, for purposes of this explanation, that person A will share, person B will listen. A shares what she is feeling, but only one statement at a time. B hears each statement and responds with only the phrase, "Thank you." The "thank you" is simply to acknowledge that A's communication has been received. The listener may have difficulty with the limited response. We are so used to first mentally rehearsing our judgments and comments that the urge to say more may be great. It is important to use only the "thank you" and no more in order that the speaker receive complete attention. A shares with B all of her present or conscious past feelings of the day (or before if necessary) for up to ten minutes. B responds to each feeling with a "Thank you," until A feels finished.

Then B takes a turn sharing in the same procedure. A may respond with only the same "Thank you," and no more. B completes the exercise or shares for ten minutes. When the sharing is complete, each person can take a moment to thank the other for sharing in a way that respects both, perhaps a kiss, a hug, or just a glance.

It is not fair to say things like "I feel that you are a jerk." This is not a feeling and does not constitute a communication. "I feel hurt," however, may be more correct. It is not fair to criticize the other's communication. If A says, "I feel afraid of giving birth," B should not ask, "Why?" even after the exercise is complete.

Listen Without Rehearsing

The purpose here is to improve communication skills through what Tom Gordon (1974) of parent effectiveness training calls "active listening." Active listening is a positive, loving acknowledgment of the other person's worth. As simple as this exercise may seem, it may make the difference between a team effort that produces a relaxed labor through communication and support or a lonely, painful labor resulting from disharmony and relationship miscommunication.

Couples exchange energies in many ways. All of these exchanges are brought to the birth. Deciding what energy you would want your child born into in a conscious way may help a couple clear up the disharmony in the relationship.

Ina May Gaskin (1977) has reported on varieties of communications styles:

> Some couples exchange energy by loving, and some do their main energy exchange by fighting. One couple I know got together in an interesting way. They noticed that whenever they get near each other, they usually end up in an argument. They seemed to like to exchange energy with each other even if it was by hassling. They soon noticed that their arguments were of no consequence, so they decided they would try exchanging energy in a friendlier way and see what that was like.

Support

Support has also been eloquently described by a childbirth assistant as follows:

> Be tantric [telepathic in the language of touch] with your lady—be subtle enough in touch with her that when she tries to steer, you feel it and follow her like a good horse follows a rider. Try to do it with her exactly as she directs on the more subtle planes. If you do that, she'll trust you and get high. It's a tasty yoga—you just have to work at it, but you can do it. It's actually fancier than just dancing by yourself. You feel somebody else and let them direct; and if you let them direct, they'll tell you what to do.

Support Is Unconditional Love

Stephen wrote this account of support in *Spiritual Midwifery* (Gaskin 1977) in an attempt to convey the necessity of genuine support, without pride or ego demands that pretend that one person could even know what is right for another. High-quality support is not agreement, advice, or help. Agreement means that two people have the same ideas about a given topic or feeling. A couple might agree on common foods while shopping in the supermarket or might agree that they want to have children. Agreement sometimes passes for support. For example, adolescence is a time of great experimentation with the "forbidden," such as sex, alcohol, cigarettes, or drugs. Most of us would agree that we would prefer our teenagers not to take up smoking, drinking, drug abuse, or some (maybe any) sexual experimentation. If we have raised our children on agreement, we will withdraw our "love," because in this system it is not possible to support people we do not agree with. Their behaviors do not agree with us, so we withdraw much-needed support and may create unwanted conflict and alienation. Because support is greater than agreement, adolescents can be supported and loved even when they are doing things we do not approve of.

Labor and delivery are very activating times. Agreeing on what each feels, thinks, or wants to do may prove difficult. Support can carry a couple through these times.

Support Assumes Competence

Support is not help. There are times when help is useful and perhaps required, such as help moving furniture or help with a homework assignment. A laboring woman may need help getting out of a car or supporting her body during a contraction. However, she may not need help breathing through a contraction or handling the accompanying emotions. Such unnecessary "help" may prove to be debilitating during a time when support and self-reliance are imperative.

Gayle Peterson (1981) writes, "It is possible to accept support and help from others while maintaining independence and self-reliance. Labor is a good time to accept others' support and help. This is not always true. Some women need to experience their own strength during labor and to be alone."

One couple shared the following example of unwanted help that became a source of resentment for months after the birth. Julie and Rich learned the panting and huffing style of breathing in preparation classes. They were trying very hard throughout the labor to practice breathing and relaxing, and to really do things right. Rich wanted to be the best possible father and coach during the birth. Throughout the first stage, Julie and Rich worked well together. Then Rich became increasingly anxious and fearful that he was not doing enough to help Julie, because she seemed to be feeling so much pain. Although Julie was not asking Rich to do anything different, Rich felt that he should try harder in his role as coach. He began to "help" Julie by breathing faster and harder in her face. He kept telling her, "Breathe, breathe, breathe." The nurses joined Rich in the coaching, out of their own good will and desire to help. Julie's contractions became very intense and it was time to push. She was too involved to stop the unwanted "help" until after her daughter was born. She said she felt like a horse being cheered to victory rather than a woman giving birth. She really never communicated the upset to Rich because she "didn't want to hurt his feelings."

Ten months later, Rich ran in a local town race. It was his first race and he was very excited about putting into practice his months of jogging and speed work training. He had never run ten kilometers before. Although he heard the course was tough, he felt confident that he could do it. Julie had also been jogging some and decided to run the last mile with Rich as a way of supporting him.

At the beginning of the last mile, Rich was exhausted and very pale but still moving. Julie became anxious that he would not make it and wanted to help Rich finish. She started to coach him in longer, deeper breaths. Rich was angry and said, "I don't need directions in how to breathe." At first, Julie was insulted, but then she remembered the birth scene.

After the race, Julie told Rich about how angry she had been at him for trying to help her breathe at the birth and how she could now understand why he had done it. She felt the inadequacy of not being able to do more, and the violation of someone trying to offer unwanted help.

Support Assumes Inner Wisdom

Finally, support is not advice. Advice, like help, is sometimes given when it is unwanted and unneeded. DelliQuadri and Breckenridge (1979) describe pregnant women as the most "well-advised" group in the culture. This advice is often the product of personal experience, and most of the time it is unsolicited.

The drama triangle can again serve as a model of this point. Every drama, remember, has three roles: Rescuer, Persecutor, and Victim. In life, these roles have a legitimate, appropriate use. Muriel James, in *Born to Win* (James & Jongeward 1973), makes the following useful distinctions.

Legitimate roles:

A persecutor is someone who sets necessary limits on behavior or is charged with enforcing rules such as a policeman or district attorney.

A rescuer is someone who helps a person who *is functioning inadequately* to rehabilitate himself such as a firefighter who carries a child from a burning building.

A victim is someone who is unjustly denied a right because of something he or she is helpless to change at that time such as job discrimination for racial reasons.

Illegitimate roles that lead to tension and drama:

A persecutor is someone who sets unnecessary strict limits on behavior or who is charged with enforcing the rules but does so with sadistic brutality such as the physician who administers Pitocin so that birth will occur before his or her weekend in the mountains.

A rescuer is someone who, in the guise of being helpful, keeps others dependent on him or her and robs the other of self-confidence such as the overly solicitous husband or nurse.

A victim is someone who pretends to need help or care and doesn't or who needs assistance but becomes dramatically helpless in order to get it such as the birthing woman who becomes a mindless "damsel in distress."

The highest forms of support may require that we keep our unwanted advice to ourselves and simply assume innate confidence in childbearing women. "Rescuer" and "persecutor" interventions negate women and rob them of their natural strength. "Damsel-in-distress" routines often elicit inappropriate and debilitating responses that further increase stress and lower self-confidence.

Be Supportable

In order to receive genuine support, it is incumbent upon laboring women to value their needs and express them clearly. Sometimes, we expect others to know what we need without our ever telling them. We even go so far as to measure another's love according to his or her ability to miraculously figure out what we want without giving them a clue. The fastest way to be robbed of self-confidence and to become a damsel in distress is to keep needs a secret and make someone else work hard to figure them out.

Support is not discouraging, demanding, criticizing, or belittling. It does not threaten, nor does it punish or abuse. True support creates a harmonious energy between partners that should not be interrupted by unnecessary outside interferences, including unneeded machinery. Sheila Kitzinger (1981) says that sometimes hospital technology can cause couples to lose their connection. She reminds us to stay in the process of support:

Men who have been giving good support to their wives before equipment is used, sometimes give up when they feel the machinery has taken over. . . . The man should not forget that however sophisticated the machinery, it is she who is having the baby. Once labor is underway, his attention should be on her, and encouragement by word, touch or look, be given with every single contraction.

Postpartum support gives couples an opportunity to practice "unconditional love" and "total positive regard," as Eric Berne (1972) and Carl Rogers (1961) taught. Genuine acceptance for who we are without our accomplishments and achievements is a rare experience in our "do-to-be-loved" culture. Such high-quality support can help prevent couples from measuring their self-worth according to their childbearing experiences and allow men and women to see their genuine, positive strengths and gains.

Touching

The importance of touching has been discussed in the previous chapter as it relates to the father's role and in the next chapter as a means for postpartum physical healing and psychological adjustment. The relationship revival requires touching as a constant source of contact, communication, and affection. Since touching and sex are so connected in the Western mind, it is important to remind ourselves that sex is a wonderful form of touching. There are countless other forms as well. This is a particularly important distinction during pregnancy, when many couples carry fears of damaging their unborn child through sexual intercourse. The mind sometimes expands this fear into anxiety over making any physical contact.

Sensitivity to Each Other

Gayle Peterson (1981) recommends touch as a means of being tender and maintaining open doorways of communication which are important in labor and in life. In her words:

> Sensitivity to touch is taught early as a means of communicating to the laboring woman. Learning what she means when she says "firm" or "soft" can be discovered now. In addition to touch and massage as a means of labor support, it is important for the woman to learn to touch her husband or labor support person. In this way, she can learn how to better communicate her own preferences.

Touching during pregnancy not only aids in maintaining closeness, but also can prepare couples for labor by improving their touch awareness.

Eric Berne (1972) referred to "touch" as a hunger. In fact, he noted the work of René Spitz, who observed institutional infants who lacked the physical support of touching and cuddling. They became physically deprived and slowly lost their appetites, a condition that improved almost immediately with the help of volunteer "mothers" who touched the children daily. A well-known bumper sticker that says, "Have you hugged your child today?"—with variations including your teacher, nurse, and lawyer—reminds us of the need to touch and be touched.

There are several materials that suggest touching exercises during pregnancy, including *Birthing Normally* (1981) by Peterson and *The Experience of Childbirth* (1981) by Kitzinger. Other manuals on touch and massage may provide additional ideas and techniques. Before a couple engages in touching, it is important to remember to touch from a place of love and caring. Doing a touching exercise because one *should* is probably the fastest way to dissipate intimacy and to increase resentment. It is useful to allow lots of psychological room for spontaneity and natural expression, without trying too hard to get the desired results. The purpose of this section on touching is to serve as a reminder, a consciousness raiser to couples regarding the value and need for touching in life and in childbirth.

Release Psychological Stamps That Prohibit Touching

Occasionally couples collect resentments and forget to share them. Transactional analysts refer to this as stamp collecting, borrowed from the practice of collecting supermarket stamps that can be pasted in a book and later redeemed (Berne 1972). Stamp collecting in relationships refers to the psychological accumulation of hurt or anger or other feelings that are stored until one is justified in dumping them. Sondra Ray's (1980) warnings of the effects of withheld feelings include the following: "First of all, your body will be in pain if you are withholding communication; second, the other person will become confused; third, the relationship will get crazy."

Withholding the truth about feelings is often translated into withholding of physical touch and affection. Attempting to touch or exchange physical contact when partners are withholding hurt may lead to further upset. The following exercise is offered to couples who notice withheld resentment and desire to release themselves of it. It is offered with the caution that desiring to release oneself of emotional hurt and desiring to heal the relationship must continue to remain the central purpose. The process has the potential for becoming an irresponsible blame-game of more inflicted hurt rather than relief. When done with love and responsibility, it is a caring, opening exchange that has proven effective in clearing up the physical contact in many relationships.

Practice Touching

Find a quiet time when each person has adequate physical energy and emotional investment in the process. Find a place where you will not be disturbed or distracted by outside influences. Sit quietly, across from each other, with knees touching and eyes closed, for about three minutes—to relax the body and calm the mind.

Reread the communication process for more detail if needed. Then, gaze into each other's eyes as a reminder of your commitment to yourself to engage in this process from a loving, caring place. Choose who will share first, herein referred to as *A*. *B* will be the listener, and will also assist *A* by asking *A* the following question: "What are you withholding?" *A* responds with one statement, such as, "My fears about the baby," or, "My anger at you for working late last week." *B* responds with, "Thank you," and no more, and then asks the same question again: "What are you withholding?" *A* responds, and this sequence is repeated until *A* can honestly say that he or she is no longer withholding anything that he or she is aware of at that time.

Then the couple switches roles, engaging in the same procedure until *B* is able to arrive at the same conclusion. Sometimes the person sharing may feel blocked and unable to think of a response. The listener should allow a few moments of silence and then say, "Thank you," even if nothing is spoken. The silence is often an attempt to communicate an item not fully known to the conscious mind.

When this procedure is finished, the partners close their eyes and take a moment to reflect on the experience. Then, with open eye contact, *A* says to *B*, "I forgive you and me for everything. I love you and me completely." *B* repeats the same phrase. The partners take time to thank each other for sharing. If future resentments arise, repeat the exercise. Remember not to do it while taking care of children, driving in the car, or involved with some other distraction. Success depends on mutual commitment and intention for resolution.

Once withheld feelings are expressed, once withheld touch is more easily and spontaneously expressed, couples who develop such a structure for handling upsetting feelings increase their chances of having a satisfying, joyful childbirth, free of the baggage of past hurts and open for the new life ahead.

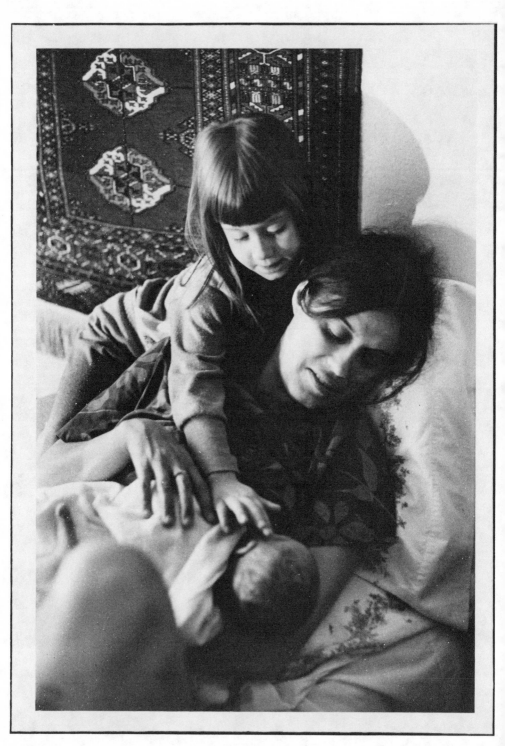

10

Postpartum Expression

In order for the mother to be born, the pregnant woman must die. The inner sanctum that once protected and nurtured fetal life collapses, returning the body to its former, nonpregnant state. A pregnant woman is a symbolic representation of motherhood, family, strength, vulnerability, femininity, and more. Very few feel neutral toward this emotionally activating symbol, and she tends to attract much emotional support and advice.

Male partners generally feel more protective, affectionate, and attentive. They are likely to feel manly, grown-up, and fatherly in her presence. They are more apt to bring flowers, do housework, and help with other children at this time.

About-to-be grandparents are more likely to call, to write, or to become reinvolved in their children's lives. They more easily drop old conflicts and complaints and update their relationships with their offspring to produce more adult-to-adult communication.

Friends and relatives often have parties in honor of the pregnant couple and their expected child, literally "showering" them with gifts. As Bittman and Rosenberg Zalk (1978) write of expectant fathers in the first trimester, "Those who love him will love him more." The phone will likely ring more often and the couple will receive special considerations in the planning of events and at social gatherings.

Even strangers smile, help the pregnant woman on and off buses, and offer to carry her bags. They open doors, begin conversations, and express congratulations. The spirit is almost pre-Christmas—when the world is celebrating, giving and sharing in honor of birth. In short, the pregnant woman is often the focus of much ado. For some women this time may serve to heal a history of loneliness, isolation, and a lack of family contact. For others, it may be a delightful serendipitous gain. For all women, these responses are suddenly and substantially altered at birth or shortly after.

The Postpartum Attention Shift

Just as the Christmas spirit fades with the coming of the new year, the liberating permission to be open, offered by the presence of the pregnant woman, disappears with the pregnancy. Male partners shift some of their protective urges and attention toward children. Mothers also shift from their primary focus on the spouse to the encompassing care of a child.

Grandparents still call and drop by, but with greater interest in the new grandchild than in the parents. They may even demonstrate a kind of unconditional love and affection toward their grandchildren that is not burdened with the parental guilts, demands, and judgments that they felt toward their own children. Grandparents may love our babies the way we ourselves always wanted to be loved.

Friends and relatives also visit, bringing gifts and flowers in booty-shaped pots, and spending more time in the presence of the newborn than with the parents. Strangers are less friendly. Ironically, women report that fewer doors are opened when the baby (and accompanying paraphernalia) is carried in the arms than when the baby was in the uterus. The phone rings less often and the baby demands more. Like the passing of Christmas with the "holiday blues," pregnancy yields to birth and then to the natural healing process commonly called postpartum depression.

Although the process itself is natural in its essence, it is culturally influenced and is psychologically as well as physiologically upsetting. It has been thought that women experience postpartum depression because of the intense and rapid hormonal changes of childbearing. It is true that great stress is placed upon the physiologic stamina of the mother. As Helene Deutsch (1945) notes, "The organism no sooner recovers from the great physiologic shock of delivery than it must assume a new physiologic function, suckling the child." However, the psyche must also adjust, and it is not reacting just to hormonal imbalances and readjustments. A study in the *American Journal of Psychiatry* by Asch and Rubin (1974) revealed that both fathers and adoptive parents undergo a postpartum adjustment and emotional upheaval as well, underscoring the normal psychological postpartum stress.

Grief for What Is Lost

Postpartum depression is actually a grief reaction to loss—to the loss of the baby within; the protective and affectionate emotional responses; the dreams of returning to childhood; the special considerations and courtesies;

the intimate one-to-one relationships with partners; and so on. The transition from pregnancy to parenthood produces natural stress accompanied by unavoidable emotional loss.

Delliquadri and Breckenridge, in their book *Mother Care* (1979), refer to the fifteen years of clinical experience of Dr. Bertram Cohler. He concluded in a conference presentation in 1977, "Only sudden death of a loved one is as stressful as the birth of a first child, and the depression, grief and mourning women undergo after giving birth is understandable." The authors go on to outline a psychological basis for understanding the process of postpartum and some hints for good "mother care" that truly supports the concept of positive birthing.

Heal Thyself . . . Then Bond

There is much pressure on the educated Western woman to respond to her infant in the "right" way after birth. This point was made in an earlier chapter, but it is worth repeating. The bonding studies of Klaus and Kennell (1982) revealed the positive results of early maternal-infant contact and proclaimed a critical time frame in which this contact was optimal. However useful this information has been, it has also led parents to believe that failure to bond within this critical time frame produces unhealthy parent-child relationships as a result of some permanent loss. This notion has led many parents (especially mothers) to unnecessary guilt and mental anguish when they were too exhausted from labor to really feel like bonding or were separated from their infants because of some hospital policy or actual emergency. The damage done is not in the lack of bonding, which takes place gradually over several months, but in the mental anguish suffered over believing that psychological damage has been done.

Cultural Lack of Support

Professor Conrad Arensberg has coined the term "matrescence" for the period during which a new mother slowly grows comfortable with her baby and her new role as mother (Raphael 1973). American mothers are expected to achieve full matrescence sooner than anywhere else in the world. Mothers are usually on their own upon leaving the hospital a few days after birth. Dana Raphael (1973), anthropologist and author, points out that the transition to matrescence is much more gradual in non-Western cultures, where the new mother is eased into motherhood—where she is forbidden to work, lift, or cook, is fed special foods, and is sung to and often even held and rocked just as she holds and rocks her new baby.

In addition to undergoing the physical reorganization of her body, the normal depression of postpartum grief, and the pressure to respond as an effective parent without previous training, the postpartum woman is likely to attempt these adjustments while spending much time alone. Judith Duncan (1982), in a paper presented at the 1982 Perinatal Social Workers Conference, described postpartum women with normal healthy babies as the loneliest group in the country. They are "unfortunate" enough to have birthed healthy babies and therefore are not expected to need special services, nor will they receive any. Perhaps this isolation accounts for the depth of depression sometimes experienced by Western women. From the onset of pregnancy, there are cultural variations in women's responses, both physiologically and psychologically. Western women often complain of nausea, a very real and debilitating experience at times. Physicians tend to treat nausea as a foregone conclusion and may casually prescribe Benedictin, even though the drug is under suspicion and may be dangerous. Yet, in other cultures where the pregnant woman is revered and respected, nausea may be nonexistent. In some societies of New Guinea, Margaret Mead found no nausea, but rather pregnant women erupted with boils in the first trimester and proudly displayed them as a symbol of their pregnancies (Kitzinger 1980).

Postpartum Expression Honoring the New Mother

A woman's postpartum reactions change just as dramatically from culture to culture. In her book *The Tender Gift: Breastfeeding* (1973), anthropologist Dana Raphael contrasts postpartum experiences in other cultures with our own. The Ticopia of the Solomon Islands announce the birth of a child by saying, "A mother has given birth!" rather than," A child is born!" This announcement is symbolic of the reverence and respect given to the postpartum mother. While the child is jubilantly welcomed, the new mother is tenderly cared for. This culture (and most of the other 250 cultures Raphael studied) believes that the mother's well-being and good health is of paramount importance so that she can successfully nurture her child. The mother is fed, cared for, and coddled, a custom consistent with Janov's belief that women psychologically relive their personal birth experiences during childbirth and therefore need special care in the postpartum weeks.

The new mother among the Ticopia is assigned a *"doula,"* a woman who will help, counsel, encourage, and support her. Postpartum depression is unknown. Contrasted with the Western woman, who is expected to be awkward, nervous, routinely depressed, and unsupported, the Ticopia woman is expected to receive special attention for as long as it is needed in an atmosphere of dignity and respect.

British anthropologist and author Sheila Kitzinger (1981) believes that much of our postnatal depression is a result of Western childbearing practices. She believes that women, who want only to be with their newborns in a process of getting to know them and growing comfortable with them, are demoralized by the efficient and well-meaning hospital staff who take over the infant's care and leave the mother feeling as though the baby belongs not to her, but to the hospital. Although this explanation accounts for only a part of the postpartum adjustment process, Western birth modes that still separate mother and child may activate maternal loss feelings unnecessarily and certainly add to the depressive reaction.

Since most of us will probably not move to the Solomon Islands to give birth, we will probably experience postpartum reactions in some form. A few rare women may avoid the postpartum emotional upheaval, but most of us will not, and we therefore need the best information and self-acceptance possible. Many women have reported to us experiencing let-down, left-out, lonely feelings after birth. Yes, normal changes are present as mentioned earlier, but there is much more to postpartum reactions than just hormones and belief systems within Western culture. Perhaps with an adequate understanding of the grieving process and an attitude of maternal well-being as the primary goal, postpartum depression could become postpartum expression—a time when women could express their feelings, needs, and wants in an atmosphere of acceptance and care such as that offered by the Ticopia.

Health in Depression—A Sign to Rest

In his book *Depression and the Body* (1972), Alexander Lowen described depression as a time of healing and as a natural state of recuperation after an expenditure of energy or stress. In this sense, postpartum reactions are healthy responses that signal the body to rest and the mind and emotions to recover. The healing process is a total one involving the body, mind, heart, and soul.

In earlier chapters, birth was described as stress, normal stress. Stress throws the body out of balance. It may lower the immune system and create vulnerability to disease or infection. In cases of serious physical loss such as miscarriage, stillbirth, or infant death, women may experience prolonged stress that may become a precondition for cancer.

In cases of normal postpartum grieving, the stress is less severe and is likely to make the body more vulnerable to colds, sinus infections, and sore throats, which might have the psychological interpretation of withheld tears. One couple reported that between the two of them, they contracted seventeen separate colds and infections during the first postnatal year. The illnesses were compounded and prolonged by lack of sleep, but were believed to be part of their postpartum adjustment. They each reported feeling tremendous needs for physical care such as massages, touching, and special foods, but did not know how to ask for it without being sick. Once they expressed their anger and sorrow and losses from childbirth on, and learned to communicate their physical needs, they were able to spend the second postnatal year free of infection—even with continued limited sleep.

Simple Healing Aids

Physical touching is a primary healing force. As previously mentioned, our physical touching is all too often confined to sexual foreplay and actual intercourse. With a postpartum ban on sex, postpartum couples starving for physical support may wait weeks or months to engage in touching. In sections of India, women are routinely massaged for days and even weeks after birth, and show very few signs of depression as we know it. Surgically delivered and medically interrupted women are even more desperate for touch because of the unavoidable violations to the physical body and the accompanying breakdown of the etheric field, the invisible outer protective energy surrounding the body.

Foods for recuperation and the nutritional needs of nursing also aid in the recovery of the body. All too often, the postpartum mother finds no time to cook for herself as she attempts to meet the demands of her infant. Friends and family who want to support should be given recipes and designated cooking days to free new mothers of this undue burden and to provide much-needed nutritional aid. Although women are often programmed not to be burdensome and to refrain from expressing their needs, postpartum women need help and support in *expressing* rather than *depressing* that need.

The Postpartum Mind and Heart

The mind begins to prepare for postpartum reactions during the last trimester, and especially during the last month, by regularly running mental movies of the events to come. These mental movies, however, are often inadequate representations of the realities of post-birth. Studies previously mentioned indicate that childbirth preparation falls short of adequately preparing a couple for transitions to parenthood, and, therefore, many couples have not adequately mustered available resources in anticipation of the events to come. They are not aware of the mind's capacity to store loss-related events that may be reactivated in postpartum weeks and months. The natural losses that accompany childbearing were described at the beginning of this chapter. These losses exist in each parent in some form and will pass according to one's capacity to understand and respect grief. It is important to know that previous losses may be reactivated at this time, especially if the emotional charge associated with the prior loss has been withheld. The most common example of postpartum activations of the past is found in women who have lost their mothers before becoming mothers themselves, even if the actual loss occurred years ago. There is a natural tendency to feel connected with our mothers during the childbearing process and to grieve in their absence, as expressed in Colleen's report.

Colleen's Story

My son was born after a normal eight-hour labor at a community-based hospital. My husband and I were very pleased with the birth. Labor went well and the hospital staff were wonderful. They were all on my team. Matthew, our son, was just beautiful. He was over 8 pounds and really awake. I held him for hours after birth and didn't want to give him up. I actually fell asleep with him in my arms and my husband at my side. We left the hospital three days after the birth and went home to several relatives and friends who'd prepared a wonderful brunch. It was then that I first began to notice my mother's absence. It was strange to think of her since she had actually died almost twenty years ago when I was 13. She'd been somewhat sickly for a few years before her death, but I didn't know she was so seriously ill with cancer until about a month before her death. Her room smelled so strong I was afraid to go in to see her. It seemed like we grew apart even though I knew she still loved me. When she died, my older sister took over. Things were never the same, and I always wanted my mom to come back. I'd dream about her and imagine that she was going to be just outside my door some morning. Of course, she never was.

A few weeks after Matthew's birth, I began to dream about my mother again. I didn't really connect the dreams to anything but I was very anxious and depressed. For many weeks, I thought I was just having "baby blues" that would go away any day. I knew I was lonely and tired. Things got worse. I felt crazy, like I wasn't handling things well. I didn't want to tell anyone because I thought I was sort of weak for not being able to pull myself out of the pits.

Finally, I called my doctor who brushed me off at first, but I insisted on some kind of help even though I didn't tell him how desperate I really was. He referred me to my counselor. I felt bad about having to go because it seemed like another sign of my inability to handle things myself. Once I got some information about what was happening to me, I started to feel normal again. I could see how angry I was at my mother for dying and how much I wanted her to be around for Matthew's birth. It took me a few weeks to forgive her. When I did I noticed that there were many people who wanted to support me but I'd rejected them because they weren't my mother. Once I started accepting help, the depression and anxiety disappeared. It was such a relief to have the energy to take care of Matthew

*because on top of everything else I was feeling awful because I really didn't
have the energy to be a good mother.*

Other Losses Recalled

Loss is probably one of our first life experiences. If a grieving parent is
confronted with a large stack of unexpressed, unresolved losses, the impact
is intense, but the opportunity for much healing is equally great. It is
impossible to know exactly what is stored in our mental file cabinets. The
point is that each mind is a unique system and each parent's postpartum
period is a unique process, one that deserves our highest respect.

Sharing of feelings and thoughts is a key to peace of mind. Our mental
tapes can cycle in a closed loop system without relief unless they are released
through verbal sharing. As family members may also be activated, outside
listeners offering genuine support can be very helpful.

Stages of Grieving

Most experts have defined the emotional aspects of grieving according to
stages or phases. Since postpartum is a time of healthy grieving, it is not
unusual for the postpartum parent to pass through some or all of these
phases. Although some possible reactions will be outlined here, it is more
useful to remember the unique, individual process within than to slot ourselves into a category or to look for a road map for perfect postpartum
expression. It is also more useful to focus on developing healthy, effective
styles of grief expression than to be concerned about doing it correctly.

Elements of Grieving

There are five common experiences associated with grieving.

DISBELIEF

The first stage is one of disbelief, a time of mental shock, as the events
of birth bring about rapid changes. Most parents attending our seminars
reported some sense of disbelief or numbness just after birth. However,
very few viewed this reaction as normal, and they were afraid that they
were somehow failing at bonding or were being unloving toward their children. One father said he felt as if he floated out of his body. His face was
smiling. He was holding his baby. He knew he was proud, but did not have
any emotions or body sensations to validate the experience.

ANGER

Anger is characterized by feelings of frustration, irritation, envy, and blame. Kitzinger refers to these normal postnatal feelings in her work *The Experience of Childbirth* (1981). She says, "The mother—even though she hesitates to admit it—often harbors a secret resentment against the baby who has deprived her of her freedom. . . . The mother's secret resentment of the baby can be further exaggerated by the husband's jealousy of his child." Anger is probably one of the most difficult feelings for the postpartum couple to express. Often resentment is withheld because of fear that the infant will be damaged in some way or will feel unloved. The irony of this belief is that the greatest damage is always done when resentment is withheld rather than expressed between two supportive, communicating adults.

One couple shared at a seminar an anger toward each other and their child that was manifested every Saturday afternoon. Before they became parents, both worked full time in busy jobs that demanded much of their time. On weekends, they would often spend Saturday in bed watching monster movies on television as a form of relaxation. After their child was born, they still sat in front of the television on Saturday afternoons trying to recover the lost intimacy and freedom resulting from parenthood. For weeks, they watched parts of monster movies in between the crying or babbling of the baby, ending the afternoons in anger, which often turned into an argument. Once they could express their natural feelings with self-acceptance, they stopped trying to regain the past and started finding new ways to spend Saturday that were far more satisfying and conducive to family life.

GUILT

Western parents are programmed to feel guilty even before conception. We are guilty for what we do, what we eat, what we do not do, what we do not eat, what we say, what we do not know, what we feel, what we do not feel, and so on and so on. We blame ourselves for our children's behavior, grades, skinned knees, and bumped heads. Although it is probably quite impossible to escape guilt in pregnancy, childbirth, and postpartum, minimizing self-punishment and gathering accurate information can lead to much liberation from guilt. Expressing fears, asking questions, and seeking support are useful actions against guilt and support postpartum *expression*.

DEPRESSION

Depression is a frightening word in Western systems with which normal reactions are easily translated into psychiatric disorders. Depression is a healthy reaction to stress and a signal for the need to recuperate. It is successfully managed when we, especially as women, do not become victims of our depression. Inner childhood messages that define women as damsels in distress or forbid them to be burdensome cause us to become victims and therefore prolong depression.

The scripting patterns that create helplessness were previously discussed. These patterns cause women to lose focus on their needs and to become sick, overwhelmed, and distraught in order to receive assistance. A similar result also occurs in women who have become overly independent as a style of coping with today's sexism. Colette Dowling, in *The Cinderella Complex* (1981), calls this reaction the counterphobic style. T. Berry Brazelton, in *On Becoming a Family* (1981), writes, "Most women want to be pampered, to be taken care of during childbirth and the following days. They might not like to admit a longing for dependency, and it may be harder for a woman who has been successfully independent before." It is often difficult for women to surrender to depression when pathological diagnosis looms just around the corner and when treatment may be severely inappropriate. Although most women have probably not experienced the extreme mishandling of Emily and David, their story serves to make the point.

After their first child's birth, Emily felt joy and euphoria. Then, the early excitement was overshadowed by fear, fatigue, and depression. David was unprepared, bewildered, and worried about his wife, as well as coping with his new fatherhood. For Emily, the depression was intense and evoked physical symptoms such as chills and tremors, all normal grief reactions according to Peppers and Knapp, authors of *Motherhood and Mourning: Perinatal Death* (1980). Her doctor recommended hospitalization, which turned into a psychiatric workup. Emily writes:

> I've always felt that if they let me express all the "crazy" thoughts and feelings I'd had when I arrived, I'd have been better off. Instead, I was given a drug that shut everything off and had horrible side effects. I finally left the hospital (against medical advice) and took myself off the drugs. Not taking them gave me back enough of myself to know they were not good for me. Even so, it took me another ten full days to cry.

In order that others may not suffer the unnecessary pain and bewilderment of Emily and David, we as women must value our psychological process and refuse systems that promote further pain. Let us begin to understand the reality of postpartum depression in order that we may begin to foster postpartum expression.

ACCEPTANCE AND ADJUSTMENT

The last experience in grieving is acceptance, which leads to successful adjustment. This is the passageway to successful family living, although it may not be a happy time. Here conflicts are settled, feelings expressed, and appropriate adjustments made. The movie-watching couple, who were angry at their loss of freedom and intimacy, expressed their anger, accepted their roles as parents, and began to plan Saturday afternoons as a new family. Acceptance, not with resignation but rather with maternal well-being, leads to successful future family living. As DelliQuadri and Breckenridge write in *Mother Care* (1979):

> With all the changes you must face in the first months of parenthood—shifts in your family responsibilities, the time you can spend together, even in your sexuality—don't be discouraged if your adjustments seem to be taking time. You have many years ahead of you, as parents and as lovers.

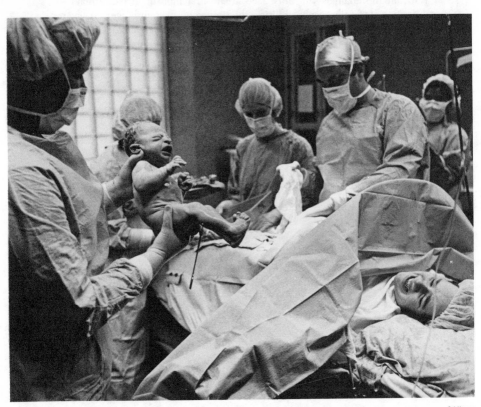

11

Cesarean Deliveries: Psychological Healing & VBAC Preparation

The status of Cesarean deliveries in our country today is the source of much heated debate among medical professionals and also of rising consumer concern. Only fourteen years ago, the Cesarean section rate was 5 percent of all births. Today, that figure has more than tripled. In some large urban teaching hospitals rates as high as 35 to 50 percent are common (Cohen & Estner 1983).

In 1979, Helen Marieskind reported to the Department of Health, Education and Welfare that the most frequent reason given by obstetricians for increased Cesarean rates was "threat of malpractice," although studies of insurance claims do not seem to justify this fear. In "An Evaluation of Cesarean Section in the U.S.," she reported that automatic repeat Cesarean (about 30 percent of all Cesareans annually, somewhere between 200,000 and 250,000) was the second most frequent reason stated by obstetricians. This reason also seems to lack validity. In fact, Marieskind estimates that over $90 million may have unnecessarily been spent by insurance companies in 1979 alone, due to the procedure of automatic repeat Cesarean. Nancy Cohen and Lois Estner (1983) reviewed the studies of vaginal birth after Cesarean and discovered that *no study since 1930 has proved vaginal birth after Cesarean harmful.* In fact, most studies suggest strong uterine dependency and probable success for many women.

The American College of Obstetricians and Gynecologists (ACOG) has responded to consumer pressure with a modified policy of Dr. Craigin's 1915 dictum, "Once a Cesarean, always a Cesarean." The policy calls for individual evaluation of Cesarean-delivered women but limits candidates according to birth weight and confines birthing to strict policies that pyschologically inhibit women in labor. (ACOG 1982). The changes are much needed, but there is still a chasm between the approaches of the Cesarean Prevention Movement and of ACOG.

As a result of what some have termed "surgical vandalism," consumer groups have been formed (e.g., Cesarean Education Support and Concern and the Cesarean Prevention Movement). These groups plead for conscious awareness and informed choice on the part of childbearing women and couples. Suzanne Arms (1975) writes that Cesarean deliveries may become the method of choice in the future, a suggestion not very far-fetched when you consider Brazil's Cesarean rate of 60 percent (Meyer 1979).

The men and women behind these consumer groups are attempting to awaken Western women to the many myths of natural childbirth that led to Cesarean deliveries, and to the risks involved in surgical procedures to both mother and child. The success of these groups depends on a deepening sense of confidence and focus on well-being among women. Without a strong sense of self, established medical practices cannot be effectively questioned. Angry attacks upon the system only stimulate further aggression. Angry words inappropriately expressed (even very justified emotions) elicit in return verbal weapons, knives, and machines. So it becomes increasingly important that ineffective institutional policies be confronted with information, consumer advocacy, and a positive and responsible sense of self.

In order to be truly well informed on the status of Cesarean deliveries, the politics of surgery, and the safety of vaginal birth after Cesarean, the much-cited work of Nancy Cohen and Lois Estner, *Silent Knife* (1983), and the work of New York lay midwife Lynn Richards should be read. At the time *Silent Knife* was written (1982), Ms. Cohen had personally worked with 173 women seeking vaginal birth after Cesarean and had a 91 percent success rate to that date. Future politics and medical realities of Cesarean sections are not within the scope of this book. However, individual psychological healing and a focus on positive birthing are necessary in order for the larger, institutional violations to be confronted and stopped.

The Psychological Effects of Cesarean Sections

Surgical deliveries have profound psychological effects on all women, whether the surgery is actually necessary and life-saving or not. The Cesarean mother has much added stress. Delliquadri and Breckenridge in *Mother Care* (1979) remind us that the Cesarean mother is both "postpartum and post surgical." The recovery involves body healing and emotional resolution.

This is not to discount that recent changes in Cesarean sections have made deliveries more humane and family-centered. Linda Meyer in *The Cesarean (R)Evolution: A Handbook for Parents and Childbirth Educators* (1979), describes how Cesarean women now have choices over medications, father participation, and maternal-infant separation that were once automatically regulated by hospital policies. Although these changes are helpful, there is no way to avoid the postpartum, postsurgical grieving and necessary recovery.

To say, "We had a great Cesarean!" may mean that the delivery was the best possible surgical procedure with much emotional support and caring. To imagine one has escaped psychological grief (especially in cases of unplanned Cesareans) and body violation is to be painfully and perhaps dangerously unconscious of oneself. This is not to deny or attempt to invalidate any individual experience but simply to point out the innate health and consciousness in women who notice normal postpartum stress and emotional turmoil.

The previous chapter contained a description of grieving including the necessity of physical, mental, and emotional healing. The stages of grief from shock and numbness to acceptance and hope are described in detail. This data is applicable to the postpartum Cesarean mother and father, with varying degrees of expression. Nancy Cohen and Lois Estner (1983) note that the post-Cesarean mother grieves for all the same losses as the vaginally delivered woman. They go on to say that she has the added losses typical of Cesareans, which include loss of control, of dreams, of teamwork in birth, of maternal-infant contact. These additional losses intensify and prolong the grieving process.

The Violated Body

The body always suffers violation in surgery. For example, when we go to the dentist for a filling or even a check-up, our bodies incur some minor violation. It is not natural to be numbed by the artificial chemicals contained in Novocain, to keep our mouths so open to potential bacteria, to be drilled with high-power tools or cut with small instruments. It is upsetting to be violated even for a short time. These minor violations may actually take days or weeks to heal. Many Westerners avoid dental care and chastise themselves for not going to the dentist—even though there is psychic health in avoiding the violation. However, there are times when oral health requires our willingness to submit to known violation, hopefully by caring, concerned hands sensitive to our (patients') reality.

So, with a Cesarean delivery, does the body receive artificial numbing through a spinal or general anesthesia, which is in and of itself very frightening. The surgical cutting, the tugging and pulling, as well as the exposure of vulnerable internal organs to external toxins, all violate the body. The recovery in some women takes as long as six months to a year, while her time and energy are being consciously directed toward loving and caring for her child. Many women chastise themselves for submitting to the surgery, adding greater stress to the postpartum grieving and recovery process.

Some women report that, after a Cesarean, their bodies became very sensitive to further violation. A slight bump such as a stubbed toe might be very painful. Other women may feel that their bodies "toughen" in an attempt to guard against further violation, making it difficult at times for the Cesarean mother to receive affection, have sexual intercourse and orgasm, and express her natural urges to touch those around her.

Nutritional care can aid in the physiological recovery. The immune system of the Cesarean mother is greatly strained. Actual vitamin and dietary information can be found in Linda Meyer's *The Cesarean (R)Evolution* (1979), and in Gail Brewer's *What Every Pregnant Woman Should Know* (1977), or can be obtained at local health food stores.

Occasionally, women report that there is difficulty healing the incision or pain in the lower abdomen, or both, that do not have a physiological explanation. We have discovered that this is an area of the body where women store normal anger at the violation and may feel that they are not justified in expressing it. Many women report that they feel they should be grateful, especially if they have live, healthy babies. Anger-release work followed by custom-designed visualizations often heal the lower abdomen and desensitize the violated area, making touch more pleasant.

Releasing the Emotional Charge

Expression of anger and hurt may take a variety of forms. The following are a series of letters written by one woman as a release exercise. It should be noted that expressing anger or other hurt feelings may be difficult in times of such political turmoil in the birthing field. Men and women are too often left to wonder whether the Cesarean was life-saving or not. Without taking a complacent view toward the rising Cesarean rates, it's useful to know that although not all Cesareans are necessary, they are unavoidable in the sense that each parent, each birthing woman, acts on the best information and resources available to them at the time. Expressing feelings has nothing to do with other people's competence, motivation, or caring. It has nothing to do with having faith in a doctor, a husband, or a midwife. Feelings are simply that, feelings. They do not detract from our love for our children.

In fact, it was love that allowed the Cesarean mother to surrender in surgery in the first place.

Mary Ellen's Story

Mary Ellen is a 28-year-old mother of four. Three of her children were Cesareans. Her twins were born in 1976. She and her family live in a Boston suburb and her deliveries took place at a major urban hospital in the Boston area.

> *I was surprised and upset when I was told I needed a Cesarean delivery. My labor was almost twenty-eight hours long and I felt like I was almost there. I had a monitor and was shaved, and was already feeling scared. My twin daughters were breech twins and couldn't be vaginally delivered because of their locked position. I was afraid they would die.*
>
> *I was given a large dosage of general anesthesia and was unconscious for almost ten hours. I woke up alone in the recovery room. There was a lot of noise. My body was in tremendous pain and my voice was too weak to get anyone's attention. I remember feeling so enraged that no one came to my aid.*
>
> *My daughters were not allowed to come home because they were under 5 pounds. I visited them two times a day for several hours even though I was really wiped out. I felt like a zombie walking around the hospital. I was angry to be there and angry that my body hurt so much. I loved the girls and tried not to let these feelings surface.*
>
> *I was closed off from my husband. He tried to be affectionate but I couldn't stand to be touched. He was kind but also pretty wiped out himself. I didn't have sex for almost a year. It was like I couldn't, not that I didn't want to.*
>
> *My stomach was really sore all around my incision. The area supposedly was okay but I kept imagining I had a tumor or an infection or something. Finally, I couldn't stand it.*

Mary Ellen came for counseling eleven months after her daughters were born. Over the course of six sessions she released the following in writing.

LETTER ONE: (TO MARY ELLEN'S DOCTOR)

Dear Doctor M.,
    I'm writing to tell you how much I hated being alone in surgery. It was scary and I don't know for sure what you did. I know you tied me down, I could feel it. I'm not a dog—why did you do that? I know you shaved me everywhere and made me look like a little girl and itch like crazy. I know you cut me. How can you cut people with knives? Are you a savage?

You pulled at me. I remember now. You pulled at me and at my babies. I heard your voices laughing. Am I funny? Is my body funny? What's wrong with you? I hate what you did to me.

I used to love my body. My face was never super pretty but my body was so attractive. I hate it all cut up and red. It looks awful. I don't want you to touch me or anyone to touch me. [Mary Ellen cried for thirty minutes or more at this point, when reading the letter aloud.]

I forgive you. I love my babies. I know you had to help me. I asked you to. I just had to tell you how angry I was so you could understand and I could talk to you and love my body again. Actually, I never want your job.

Thanks for listening,
Mary Ellen

LETTER TWO: (TO MARY ELLEN'S HUSBAND)

Dear Jack,

I know I am grateful to you for standing by me. Somehow—I thought you were going to protect me. It seemed like we practiced you doing the thinking and me doing the breathing. I feel angry at you for letting them cut me open, even though I don't think there could have been another way.

I wish you could know how awful it is to be cut and to have your babies tugged out. Why did you leave right after the birth? I thought you were going to stay. I thought you wanted babies and I didn't think you'd run away.

I wish I could have sex with you but I keep thinking of our babies, the birth and sex and it's all in a big ball in my head. I think I might be getting even with you for making me hurt or not protecting me from hurt. I don't want you to touch me because you didn't apologize yet. I guess you didn't know you were supposed to apologize, but you are. You are supposed to say—"Honey, I'm sorry. I didn't want this to happen."

God, I've been so hurt I couldn't see what was going on with you. We have a lot of talking to do. I didn't know it would be like this.

Love,
Mary Ellen

Unresolved Feelings May Lead to Unresolved Conflict

Mary Ellen's last letter may help to explain why some researchers have thought a possible relationship may exist between Cesarean deliveries and marital problems. Further studies indicate possible maternal-child bonding problems. It is true that maternal attachment may be interfered with by medical necessities or hospital policies that isolate infants from their mothers. It is also true that many Cesarean mothers in our seminars report an increased sense of bonding after releasing anger about the violation that was associated, as for Mary Ellen, with her children whom she so loves. This is not to accuse Cesarean mothers of child abuse but rather to point out the possible unconscious expression of feelings by women who are not supported in remaining conscious of what is happening to them, women who like Mary Ellen suffer in silence.

Since the mind tends to remember lots about our shortcomings and very little of our successes, Mary Ellen was encouraged to recall the positive aspects of her birth—which, she discovered, were many. She wrote a list of affirmations (discussed in previous chapters) and read them to herself as well:

> *I, Mary Ellen, now love my body.*
> *I, Mary Ellen, now celebrate my birth experience.*
> *I, Mary Ellen, affirm my strength and respect my feelings.*
> *I, Mary Ellen, am a very brave mother.*
> *I, Mary Ellen, am sexy and irresistible!*

Mary Ellen returned to a healthy, active sex life. She talked more with Jack and said she "fell in love" with her children all over again. Finally, after eight sessions, she reported no pain or discomfort in her lower abdomen and said that she and her husband discussed future pregnancies, reporting that they had been feeling closed to all possible options but now could more actively choose to have more children or not from a positive place.

The Loss of a Dream

Along with physical healing, the mind also seeks relief. There may be nagging questions about whether the procedure was life-saving or not and whether the couple could have done anything different. Mental questions are sometimes expressions of possible guilt feelings. It is important to get all "answerable" questions answered. It may be necessary to join consumer groups. Nancy Cohen in "Minimizing the Emotional Sequellae of Cesarean Birth" (1977) recommends referral to a local Cesarean support group which the mother can call when she needs to discuss her feelings and concerns. The mind may need to understand as much as possible about the delivery and may seek reading materials, experts, or any other source to heal itself.

The emotional process of the Cesarean couple is often one of grieving over the loss of their hopes, dreams—and, in many instances, natural ex- pectations—of natural childbirth; the loss of the teamwork and harmony of partners united in the effort to birth their child; the loss of any control in the process, and the loss of the early special moments of intimacy between parents and children. Grieving varies from person to person. Nancy Cohen and Lois Estner (1983) write that of the thousands of letters received (over 40,000), very few were written by women "feeling peaceful about their births. Most letters are filled with bitterness, frustration, confusion, sadness and pain."

Shock: May Be Due to Inadequate Preparation

Since childbirth-preparation courses usually prepare couples for hospital, vaginal deliveries, most first-time Cesarean couples are shocked, as their pictures of natural birthing are literally slashed away. Cesareans may cause couples to feel guilty, inadequate, to think that they have somehow failed. It is ironic to think that a Cesarean-delivered mother who risked her life for her child's safety could be seen as weak or inadequate. It is further ironic that women who take weeks, months, and in some cases years to recover from their surgical deliveries could think of themselves, or be thought of by others, as taking the easy way out. Yet many women and men report they do. Although they have actually done nothing that needs self-forgiveness, self-forgiveness may be a useful goal for couples who feel leftover guilt and inadequacy.

Losing control and the sense of teamwork is often another source of hurt and another loss to be grieved. Gayle Peterson in *Birthing Normally* (1981) spoke of the sense of self-confidence and psychological gain for women who actively participated in the childbirth experience. This sense is often lost by Cesarean mothers. In "Prepared Childbirth and the Concept of Control," L. R. Willmuth reported on a study in which he questioned couples to discover what factors made them feel most positive about their birth experiences. The author was able to isolate feeling of autonomy and a sense of control as being most important. Again, this sense is sometimes lost during a Cesarean.

Unresolved losses may be the source of future conflict. Accepting one's feelings and expressing them on paper or to supportive listeners, or visualizing and affirming positive living now, are keys to effective psychological resolution of Cesarean, such as that of Mary Ellen in our example.

Losing Touch with the Child

Finally, the famous work of Klaus and Kennell (1982) in identifying the instinctive, natural bonding needs in many women has further aided our understanding of the depth of grief of some Cesarean mothers who may have been separated from their babies. The urge to hold, cuddle, and touch a newborn is very strong in many parents. To be denied that urge by some life-threatening emergency, or, worse, by some *routine* hospital policy, can be deeply painful. The sorrow over not being able to have one's baby when the heart aches to parent and love is painful indeed. The long-range effects may be great unless the sorrow is released and the heart healed. As one woman wrote: "My son was fifteen before I cried about not having [had]him with me. It took us fifteen years to bond the way I wanted to. My sorrow was in the way, even though I had plenty of love to give."

Body-Mind Techniques for VBAC

This section is an overview of the psychological approach to VBAC preparation. It is included here with the understanding that not all Cesarean-delivered women are necessarily good candidates for VBAC and that some who might be will choose a subsequent Cesarean. It is written because the research supports VBAC as a physically safe and psychologically healing option for many women. The physiological and psychological impact of Cesareans is sometimes difficult to heal. VBAC, if possible, is a psychological resolution and healing in and of itself to parents who team for birthing and to women who regain faith in the functioning of their bodies. Women who seek VBAC have the right to birth their children as nature designed.

We have learned through our own seminars and through the work of Nancy Cohen and Lynn Richards that vaginal birthing has the potential to produce more emotionally satisfying birth experiences with less recovery time and more natural energy for beginning the long-awaited mother-child connection. Because recovery demands less energy, women are more able to integrate and process the experience of birth and perhaps heal any remaining emotional and, in some cases, physical conflicts.

Paula, a 30-year-old Rhode Island resident shared this letter after her VBAC birth experience. She and her husband have five children, four of whom were Cesarean delivered. The fifth birth took place at their home with much support from family and friends.

> *All during my pregnancy right up till a few days before the birth there were so many ups and downs for me. Finally I realized no matter what the odds were, what obstacles I encountered, and even what position the baby was in, I could still have a vaginal birth, it was in my power. My body could do it if I wanted it badly enough to be willing to work to achieve it.*
>
> *I have beautiful memories of my labor, although physically it was my most uncomfortable labor. I remember the quiet times of my labor, the gentleness of love that seemed to flow between Jillian and me. I'd just lie and let the power of my contractions consume me. I really enjoyed being loud at other times, singing through each contraction, I felt like I was calling to my baby to come to me, to be born. I'd get louder and louder till the contraction peaked, then I'd gently taper off. Mostly I felt comfortable to cope with labor anyway I chose to, I had support from people who loved us and I had the freedom of being in my own home. I enjoyed my labor, and even spent several hours of solitude. I watched the lunar eclipse, examined my feelings, and meditated. I felt really in tune with nature. During each contraction I did a visualization of reaching down to help birth my baby, it really opened me up, and gave such a push it was incredible.*
>
> *In the morning when Adele, Vicki and Jill arrived and my boys got up, the house was just buzzing with excitement and anticipation. Jill cooked*

everyone a big breakfast of things she brought fresh from her farm. It was like a holiday. Having our children with us was fantastic, they ran in and out of the room checking on my progress, getting wet face cloths, rubbing my back and legs. David was constantly beside me supporting and loving me. Our house was filled with so much love the day of Jillian's birth, I felt so safe and cared for. I realized this was it. I was finally going to do it, finally I was going to give birth. I could feel how strong my body was. I felt energy passing all through me. No one could stop me now, most of all no one wanted to. Pushing Jillian into the world was the ultimate experience! I felt like we were one, united, as she was moving down my pelvis. My body was doing a perfect job. My bones were even moving to make way for this little person. I was so disappointed to see only a little of her head showing. I wanted to see her. I reached down to touch her little head as it was beginning to crown and was filled with more joy than I've ever experienced in my life. I felt such a bond between us I told her, "I love you, Baby; I've been waiting for you for so long." Two contractions later David reached down to birth our daughter's body. I then lifted her on to my abdomen, and screamed, "We did it!!! (the VBAC), then announced, "We had a girl!!!"

I feel I got it all—the best that could possibly happen, a VBAC, after the four Cesareans, and a home birth at that, and a daughter after four sons. I'm still floating. My body, I love it! It's a good strong, healthy body and it's true to me. For the first time, I feel truly whole, not just because I had a VBAC but because I learned to trust my intuitions, my body's wisdom, and for the first time I really believed in myself. It took me a long time but I learned so much.

Step One: Understanding Belief

Over the past several years, we have noticed that Cesarean mothers more often report, as part of their personal history, beliefs that mentally define birth as dangerous or unsafe. They are more likely to have been the product of a difficult delivery or the focus of a family birth story that describes birth in negative and frightening ways. These thought patterns result in an instinctive urge to hold on in order to protect the child from harm. Asking parents to tell the story of their own birth or other family births or simply to express any other fears may reduce physiological tension. Dick-Read described this phenomenon many years ago in *Childbirth without Fear* (1944).

For example, Gail, a 32-year-old Connecticut mother of two, wrote, "My mother was so sick after birth and so depressed, I concluded that birth must be awful. Although she never had a Cesarean, she sure looked like she'd had more than a baby." Susan, a 27-year-old rural Californian, shared, "I remember my father telling me how lucky I was to be alive. I was born very fast and everyone always said, 'She had trouble getting started.' So did my labors have trouble getting started."

Helen Marieskind (1979) noted that women who were the most likely candidates for Cesarean delivery were primiparous (first deliveries) or multiparous (with six or more). First-time mothers were more likely than multiparous mothers to have CPD (small pelvis) or dysfunctional labor, which is usually suggestive of fear reactions, again indicating the possibility of a belief system that defines birth as dangerous.

It should be noted that Cesarean women diagnosed as CPD or dysfunctional labor are excellent candidates for future vaginal deliveries, especially when past beliefs and emotionally charged fears are released and replaced with positive, more accurate approaches to childbearing.

Cesarean mothers are less likely to have faith in their bodies and more likely to have felt critical and disapproving toward their bodies as children; these feelings are sometimes further validated by a Cesarean delivery. Nancy Cohen and Lois Estner (1983) write, "Several women with histories of infertility had very difficult births that resulted in Cesareans, although no apparent structural problems were evident. If a woman is unable to make peace with her body, normal birthing may be affected."

Marieskind's report (1979) indicated that women who had lost babies were also more likely to have Cesareans than women who hadn't, perhaps indicating further loss of faith in the physical body. Our ongoing survey at Offspring shows that women with previous miscarriages and infertility problems were more likely to be surgically delivered than women who had not. Again, these experiences point to a possible loss of faith in the physical body, and, again, a Cesarean only further confirms this psychological position.

According to other studies, couples who received the most childbirth education were most likely to have Cesareans. This validated Marieskind's conclusion that women who were the most likely Cesarean candidates were women with the most education (a 1972 survey indicated that college-educated women were the most likely Cesarean candidates) and women who had taken childbirth-education classes and expected to be in control.

These findings point to the possibility that Cesarean women place greater inner demand on themselves to be informed, well prepared, and in control. It has also been our experience that Cesarean mothers tended to seek perfectionism in themselves in many areas of their lives and had been extremely hard on themselves when goals were not achieved. This last area has been particularly useful in psychological preparation for future vaginal births, reminding us that VBAC is not the primary goal but rather is secondary to maternal well-being—mentally, emotionally, physically, and spiritually. Well-being cannot be found in perfectionistic demands, even if the goals are good in and of themselves. Physical surrender is much easier when the body's performance is not the criterion for self-love.

Lastly, there are women who believe they deserved to have a Cesarean. For example, on several occasions, sectioned mothers have shared their belief that they somehow *deserved* to be cut open in order to make up for something they felt they had done wrong, such as having had a prior abortion. Other women felt that they had to bargain with God for a live child by allowing themselves to be surgically delivered. I once heard a minister say that all God had to do was to create heaven; He could leave hell up to us. The minister was referring to our profound capacity for self-punishment.

Three important affirmations, or positive thoughts, for potential VBAC mothers are the following:

1. Birth is a completely safe experience.
2. I love my body and gain faith in it every day.
3. I deserve positive birth experiences always.

Step Two: Creating a Safe Context

Because of the fact that the obstetrical community tends to abide by the old adage, "Once a Cesarean, always a Cesarean" (a motto coined by a Dr. Craigin in 1916, when Cesarean section accounted for 1 percent of all births and was reserved for extreme cases), women and couples seeking VBAC today require much accurate data in order to make informed choices. As we go to press, a survey of twenty metropolitan Boston hospitals has indicated that *no VBAC classes are available through hospital prenatal-preparation programs*. There is a network of private instructors, however, who are affiliated with the Cesarean Prevention Movement.

It is also important to remember that most Westerners are not educated in the safety of VBAC on the basis of individual evaluations. Often, parents planning such vaginal deliveries share feelings of nonsupport from family and friends. Mothers and fathers and brothers and sisters of VBAC parents have been known to express many of the common fears and misunderstandings associated with VBAC. One woman said that her mother, upon hearing that her daughter was planning a VBAC, called her son-in-law to recommend that he make an appointment with a psychiatrist. But VBAC has been proven safe. Studies such as Cohen and Estner (1983), Douglas (1963), and Browne and McGrath (1965) all attest to the dependability of the uterus and the high likelihood of positive outcomes. Such information is essential for peace of mind.

Many potential VBAC couples feel conflict over whether to tell their own parents and families of their desire to birth vaginally. They understand that most Westerners still adhere to the old adage of chronic Cesareans rather than trust in individual evaluation. VBAC women and their partners who understand the impact of negative thinking and criticism from their own parents seek to avoid such confrontations. At times, VBAC couples in our seminars have reported lying to or distancing their own parents even though they deeply love and appreciate them, and truly want support.

It is strongly recommended that VBAC parents share their intentions as much as possible. Any lack of integrity usually produces some level of stress, regardless of our justification. However, we are the ones who must evaluate what is right and best for us. Our own inner voices must be our guides.

Finally, VBAC couples must be even more careful than others in their choice of physician and place of birthing. Since we have recognized that fearful beliefs about birth contribute to Cesarean deliveries, having a physician who is "willing to let you try" is not good enough. Old beliefs are easily activated under stress, and birthing (especally VBAC) women need more than just allowance, they need support and genuine confidence. Many hospitals still refuse VBAC mothers to use birthing rooms and consider such mothers as having a "trial of labor." The VBAC mother needs acknowledgment and support, not criticism and judgment. She and her uterus are not—must not be—on "trial."

Step Three: Affirmation and Visualization

Once the mind has been cleared of past belief patterns that create fear and tension in the body, has been given adequate information, and has been taught to accept fears as normal, it is then ready to accept new beliefs and possibilities for the future. This is done through the use of visualizations.

Affirmations are simple, positive thoughts stated in the present tense that express good ideas and beliefs. Affirmations (new thoughts) can be written, said aloud, or simply thought about repeatedly. For example, some new thoughts for VBAC couples are:

Childbirth is a safe, healthy experience.
My body is my friend and knows how to birth in my best interest.
My body labors effectively and releases my baby at exactly the right time.

Visualizations are suggested to remind women of the safety of childbirth and the effectiveness of the physical body. Visualizations are usually done on cassette tapes and are played repeatedly in order to insure positive images and relaxed bodies. Often, we suggest a potential VBAC couple's favorite music for background and ask that the couple listen to the tape at least three times a week.

The following is a sample visualization outline specifically for VBAC preparation:

Find a comfortable position in the room. You could be lying down on the floor, sitting against the wall or up in a chair. Your body should be supported in a way that requires no effort on your part. Close your eyes and just let yourself sink into the floor or chair.

Now, begin to breathe a little deeper as you let go of some of the tensions of the day. Take a deep, relaxing breath. Notice how the inhale can be used to bring in cleansing energy and how gravity is so kind that it takes the exhale away effortlessly. Notice the thoughts drifting by: thoughts about the day, this room, the future. Allow these thoughts to drift by like clouds on a windy day, weightless, effortless. It's good to have time to calm the inner being.

Inhale now with a deep cleansing breath, allowing gravity to take the exhale. As you breathe a little slower, a little deeper, allow yourself to drift off to someplace in the world or in your imagination that provides you with safety, support, comfort, and peace. Perhaps a quiet, isolated beach, or a rich green forest, or a backyard so peaceful you could hear the smallest birds sing. Wherever you go, give yourself this time to relax and settle in these beautiful surroundings.

Imagine that you or your partner is now pregnant. You may need to take special measures to insure your comfort. Take time now to bring all the necessary equipment for your total comfort—all the big fluffy pillows, chairs, hammocks, cool drinks—anything to provide total comfort. You deserve comfort and peace all the time.

Let us now begin an imaginary journey into some of the most beautiful, special parts of your body. With safety and comfort surrounding you externally, let us move to the internal, to the womb that now supports your baby with absolute strength and nourishment. Imagine this inner world: the perfect temperatures, the quieted sounds, the gentle rocking of the fetus in the protective waters. How comforting to know the body works so effortlessly to produce such perfection.

As you explore this inner world, notice the uterine walls, the lining. Send forth to these walls a healing, white light, perhaps the light of a thousand tiny angels all joining hands to guard the life within. Especially notice any areas on these walls that need special attention and send forth the healing light to provide that attention. Good.

The body has such a wonderful ability to heal itself, inside and out. Breathe and relax into the body.

Imagine now that very gently, very slowly, the body prepares to give birth. It is completely safe to imagine the body preparing for birth because the body knows when the time is right for labor to begin and no labor will begin before its time.

The preparation begins with a new flow of hormones and the slight muscular movement known as contractions. These new movements are rhythmical and increase in intensity ever so slowly, at exactly the pace that you as the birthing woman can integrate. Feel the flow of life within this womb, the muscles so lovingly working and the new meaning of pain—of health.

Notice how this baby knows to position himself or herself so that he or she too can use this little body to move with the head and shoulders toward gravity and light. Feel the power, the release of energy with each new contraction. Feel the body working so perfectly to bring forth this child.

Allow all the time you need. Let hours, days, go by, so that you and you alone are the master of this body and of this birth.

When the time is right, feel the baby entering the birth canal, inching, pushing toward the light into the gentle arms of gravity's pull.

At last, the time has come and, with a final push, the long journey is over. You see the light, feel the warm air, hear the happy voices, and rejoice in this birth. You have waited and worked so long, and now you rest, rejoice, and hold your baby lovingly in your arms.

You congratulate your body. You feel strong and capable. You know now how healthy, how naturally healing the body and mind are. You know now that all birth experiences are built on natural desires to heal, regardless of how these events appear in the external world. You take time to hold and caress your baby as long as you need.

You now have faith in yourself and in your body, knowing that this body always works in the best interest of mother and child. Because this is not the time for birth, allow your baby to reenter the womb, feet first, so that this child may be nurtured in the health of your womb. Keep in your heart the feeling of closeness, of oneness with this baby.

Slowly, bring yourself back into the room. Just begin to notice the sounds of others, the feeling of your body against the chair or floor. When you feel ready to open your eyes, you may do so, knowing that nothing will be lost. There is no scarcity of peace.

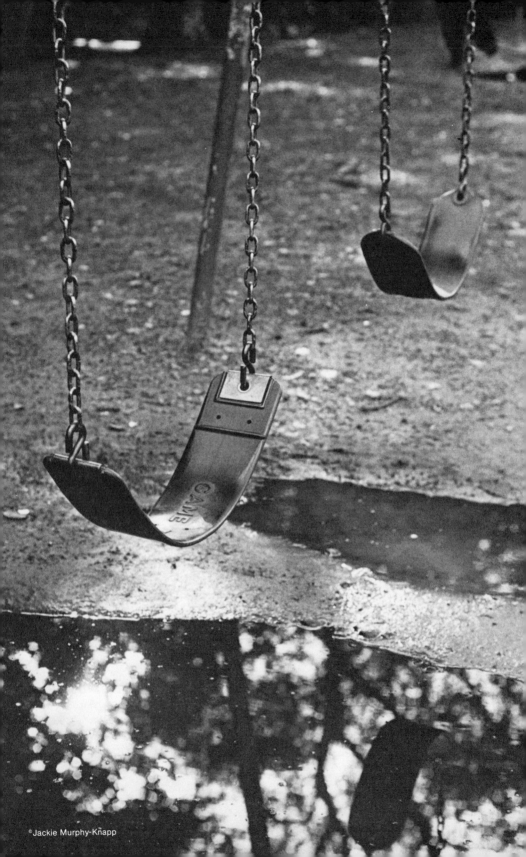

12

Ended Beginnings

Pregnancy and childbirth are the beginning of life for infants, mothers, fathers, hopes, dreams, and families. Fetal and infant loss is the end of a child's life, and the unsuspected shattering of a dream. Healing such a loss is never easy. Grief is a relentless emotion whose presence will not be evaded or denied. It is not easy to process and work through loss, to fully feel its pain, its moments of despair. Each process is unique and none deserves to be categorized, timed, judged, or criticized. Sheila Kitzinger (1981) writes, "When a baby dies, the couple lose not only the baby, but themselves as parents, and the new images of self and the other which had been built up through the months of pregnancy."

This chapter is written to assist those parents who have lost children to understand and make peace with their losses. The psychological healing of grief is very helpful in future pregnancy and childbearing. Gayle Peterson (1981) writes that when a woman experiences child-related loss, the emotional trauma is associated with pregnancy and childbirth. She says, "Mothers who have previously adopted out, or lost a baby through crib death, accident or diseases soon after birth, are often flooded with painful memories at the next labor and may require psychotherapeutic work. . ."

The topic of death in birth or pregnancy is a much-avoided subject. Very few childbirth-preparation courses discuss abortion, miscarriage, stillbirth, or infant death, perhaps because the subjects tend to bring already existing anxieties to the field of consciousness. This chapter is not an attempt to take a gloom-and-doom approach to birthing, but rather to provide a sound, realistic psychological basis for childbearing parents that may offer some a

157

much-needed opportunity to heal the past and others a reserve of information should loss be incurred.

It is true that most of the 3.5 million American women who bear children each year will give birth to healthy children who thrive and grow normally. It is always good to think positively, to believe in oneself, and to remember that chances are very good that most parents will be delighted at birth. It is also important to be able to include all possibilities, all realities, without dwelling on nightmarish fears or anxieties. Again, the process is one of release of feelings—hurt, anger, and so forth—and reintegration through visualization. It is not without pain, nor should it be without learning. Harriet Schiff opens her book *The Bereaved Parent* (1977) with a wonderful Chinese proverb: "You can't prevent the birds of sorrow from flying over your head—but you can prevent them from making a nest in your hair."

Miscarriage

Each year approximately 600,000 women miscarry in the United States alone. This figure doesn't account for unreported or unknown early miscarriages and represents 15 to 20 percent of all conceptions. This kind of loss is probably the least acknowledged and least understood of all pregnancy- and birth-related deaths. The response to the loss will vary and may include the ideas, "A miscarriage is nature's way of sparing you from having an imperfect baby"; "You can always have another baby" (Borg & Lasker 1981). In *When Pregnancy Fails*, Borg and Lasker go on to say, "These comments are heard over and over again by couples who experience miscarriage. They represent the common view that it is a minor event, or even one to be welcomed."

The Myth of Nonattachment

The idea of nonattachment is easily introduced during the first few weeks of disbelief and shock. Yet it is a painful disservice to convince oneself that miscarriage is insignificant. Peppers and Knapp, in their book *Motherhood and Mourning* (1980), noted that women grieving over miscarriage demonstrated a grief reaction equal in intensity to women grieving over fetal and infant death, different only in duration. They found guilt even greater, and the nonattachment syndrome more pronounced, in women who miscarried. Mothers who miscarry are unable to make contact with their children and are usually unable to resolve their questions and concerns about what happened. They are, rather, encouraged to forget all and go "have others." The "Pick yourself up, dust yourself off, and go get pregnant again" theme totally discounts the emotional and physical impact of the experience.

Miscarriage is death, and it demands respect, not a jocular wink and an admonition to "Go home and make a date with your husband."

The Pain of Inner Failure and Guilt

Miscarriage creates inner feelings of failure and shame, outer conflicts in marriage and family relationships, and loss of faith in the physical body. We have so much shame associated with miscarriage that we have a tradition of not sharing the news of our pregnancy with even our close loved ones until the first trimester has passed and the possibility of miscarriage diminished.

Women are already programmed to accept feelings of failure as discussed in previous chapters. With all its social secrecy, miscarriage easily activates the programmed sense of failure. Women are also programmed to carry undue burdens of guilt (sometimes called responsibility) for their children's lives, bodies, emotions, problems. When this programming is activated, it is possible to become profoundly guilty over their death even in utero.

Pizer and Palinski write, in *Coping with a Miscarriage* (1980):

> Undoubtedly, the strongest emotional response after a miscarriage is guilt. Without exception, every woman I talked with had experienced or was still experiencing feelings of guilt. They looked back for months after they miscarried, seeking a probable cause in their own behavior just prior to the miscarriage.

All losses create stress not only on the body but also on relationships. Miscarriages, like other pregnancy-related losses, are often followed by transformation for better or worse in the marriage relationship. Peppers and Knapp (1980) noted that couples tended to manifest some positive, some negative effects, but that no marriage showed no effects of a miscarriage. They particularly noted communication breakdowns among couples who miscarried, because of what they called "incongruent bonding," where the mother—having begun her attachment process—feels the significance of the loss more deeply than the father. Further, the cultural mandates for men to be cognitive and women to be emotional may leave couples in alienation and despair.

Along with possible lack of marital support, women who miscarry receive little public acknowledgment or condolences, as miscarriage is a taboo subject and is often mentioned only briefly. The body violations incurred during the D. & C. are ignored and may be further reminders of a lack of faith in the body. Women who miscarry are often a group of silent mourners, who do not feel that they qualify for support groups, yet are least likely to find emotional understanding in husband, physician, and family. When given the opportunity to release their grief, women who need to can restore faith in their bodies and can repair the psychic hurt of a miscarriage experience.

Irene's Story

———◆◆◆———

The following letter was written by a woman named Irene who discovered much unreleased anger during a grief seminar. Although she could not focus the anger on any particular person or event, she noticed that it was activated by women with small babies. Irene had had two miscarriages and was, at the time, having difficulty conceiving again. Secondary infertility is not uncommon among Cesarean women or mothers with pregnancy-related loss. Irene wrote this letter to release withheld feelings—recognizably irrational as are all feelings—but in no way pathological.

Dear Mothers of babies I don't have,

There are days when I want to walk up to you and say—"I lost my babies. Do you know what that is like?" Of course, you'd think I was crazy but I have to tell you what it's like. It's a horrible, endless nightmare. It never stops completely. When I go shopping and I hear your babies crying and gooing, I hate the sounds. I look at my groceries and think, "Where's my baby? I did all the right things."

I read books. I ate well. I rested. Yet, just when I thought I had made it past the three-month mark, I'm done in. I bleed for two days and then labor a little and then it's over. Two times in exactly the same way, I lost my babies.

I did not see them. They were too small and unrecognizable, but I knew they were gone. I know their souls, so their body formation doesn't really matter. I love them, and my husband thinks that is sick.

Your babies remind me of the hole in my belly, empty hole. The hole in my heart is probably even bigger. It's so embarrassing to face people who think you've done it and then you fail. I know my mother wants to see a baby. Look at your mothers—how alive they are when they can be grandmothers. My mother may die just a mother.

I hate being at parties where you bring your babies. I feel like a fool. I drink wine and beer but I still feel like a fool.

Some days I hate my body. I wish it worked. It just won't. Mothers, I know I must find a way to forgive myself, and then I will stop being mad at you. After today, I think I'm closer, but I might see you in a grocery store tomorrow and feel mad again. I can't tell you out loud. So I'll probably just keep writing. You see, what I really want you to know is how hurt and lonely and empty I am. I sure know.

That's all for now,
Irene

Stillbirth

Almost 200,000 women carry their babies to term or near term each year only to lose them before birth. Some labor normally and expect to see and hold a live, healthy infant. Stillbirths profoundly impact not only on the birthing woman but also men, siblings, grandparents, friends, and entire families.

In the initial shock, parents wonder whether to hold, touch, and become acquainted even for a short time with their children. Studies seem to indicate that parents who are able and are supported to make contact with their infants grieve more effectively. Dr. Emmanuel Lewis (1976), psychiatrist and author of several articles on grieving for the stillborn child, believes strongly in the concept of allowing and encouraging parents to make contact with their infants. Such contact, he feels, eases the grief process by allowing parents to grieve for someone who is more fully known to them. He further feels that, in cases of deformities, parents should not be prevented from making contact, since parents imagined mental pictures usually far worse than the actual malformation. In our own grief seminars, this has been confirmed by participants who seem to make their parent-child contact with the essence of their child, not simply the physical image. Many hospitals are now training staff members to adequately support parents with fetal and infant losses. The results reported by seminar participants seem highly encouraging.

Melissa's Story

Melissa was a 30-year-old mother who lost three children just prior to birth. The first two times, she left the hospital feeling numb and shocked, but felt anxious to get pregnant again. Her first two labors began at 6½ months, so she did not think of these as stillborns. Next, she gave birth to a healthy son, whom she viewed as a sign that her difficult times were past. Occasionally she cried, but her first two children had been "handled" by the hospital staff, without funeral services or any real acknowledgment.

Last year Melissa lost her fourth child. Again, in labor, just prior to birth. This time, however, she held her son. He was very beautiful to her. She thought of her other children, whom she had imagined as defective and malformed. She saw them in her mind as beautiful. She named her son Michael.

After his funeral, she realized that her sorrow was not only for Michael but also for her first two children, whom she hadn't named or really acknowledged. She obtained her medical records, named her children, and set up funeral services for them as well. She was finally given the external support she needed not only to accept the present but also to acknowledge the past. Each person grieves at their own pace, but there are no short cuts.

Grief for What Can Never Be

John R. Wolff and others (1970) studied the reactions of forty grieving mothers for a three-year period and noticed that significant adjustment problems were evident in all forty women (who miraculously did not develop any severe psychiatric difficulties). Others have reported evidences of grief and depression up to a year after the loss of a child through stillbirth (Jensen & Zahourek 1972).

Since grieving is a process of mourning "what is *not*," much more than a baby has been lost in a stillbirth. "What is not" is enormous. It includes not only a baby to care for and a member of a family to grow up with, but also a grandchild, a son or daughter to play ball with and shop for, the first day of school, and a "sweet 16" birthday that will never be.

A Mother Speaks

Acknowledging the depth of this loss helps to facilitate an ongoing process of release. The following is an account by a mother of a stillborn child.

At last, the day arrived when I would labor. I had waited so long. I was two weeks overdue, although I really didn't know anything was wrong. I stayed at home with my husband, Ralph, until we felt ready to go to the hospital. I was 7 centimeters dilated upon arrival and ready to go. All of a sudden—no heart beat. At first, the nurse thought I was just in the middle of a contraction, but then I was sure that something was wrong. The doctor arrived—I had never met him before. He inserted a fetal monitor and then he got a heartbeat. It was slow for a baby. Later, they realized it was mine.

"Quickly," he said. "This baby's in trouble and needs to get out!" I was wheeled rapidly down the hall—too late. My daughter did not cry. She did not move. She never breathed. I was shocked and frozen. I couldn't cry. I was just dead inside—just the way she looked. The nurses stopped speaking to me. I feel angry about that because I needed to be talked to. In fact, no one changed the dressing over my incision until a nurse from O.B. found me on the surgical ward. My incision was raw and sore. Six months later, it still hurt. The doctors were afraid to talk to me. It's funny; I never thought of suing them until they failed to talk to me.

I got pregnant five months later, and then it all hit me. I was so sad. I cried every day. I thought I was crazy and I was sure I was damaging my baby. I didn't realize that it was healthy to be so out of it. Sandra, my daughter, was on my mind all the time. It seemed like the baby I was carrying inside wasn't getting enough attention. I worried that our new baby would also die; in fact, I worried that I would kill it. Then it really hit me—how much I believed I had killed Sandra. The reports told nothing definite, but my mind believed I had murdered her somehow.

Finally, after weeks of inner torture, I decided that I'd done my best.

I don't really know why. It doesn't make a lot of sense. But I was sure glad, because I've since given birth and I'm really pleased with my son, Allan, and with myself, that we both don't have to suffer for what I couldn't have prevented.

Infant Death

There are many causes for infant death, including premature birth, congenital abnormalities, and brain damage from lack of oxygen. None of these are adequate explanations for the parent who observes a child's breath for only a few minutes, weeks, or months. The agonies of these parents include all of the physical, psychological, and emotional losses of grieving parents, but may be further burdened with questions about future outcomes, medical interventions, and life-saving procedures, as well as the nightmarish frustration of watching a child incubated and treated without being allowed to touch, hold, or console him or her.

Parents who are given a grim prognosis question whether to acknowledge their already established attachments and fear increased emotional pain by becoming further involved. As Klaus and Kennell point out in *Maternal-Infant Bonding* (1982), mothers appear to be already attached and bonded to their babies even before the children were touched or held. Following natural instincts seems to be the best guide.

Public and Personal Response

When an infant dies, public response is often awkward silence. Funeral services are usually private, and caskets are closed. Other family members do not see the lost child. One woman recently shared that she decided to allow her four children to view their brother Jonathan, who died after twenty-four hours of life. All of the children were 10 or over and had been very well prepared for the funeral service. The undertaker, however, was not, and berated the parents for opening the casket, telling them how abusive and inappropriate their behavior was.

Infant death, like other pregnancy losses, is an unconsolable loss, so friends and relatives are confronted with much helplessness and inadequacy while they mentally rehearse the "right things" to say without prescribed phrases. In an effort to avoid inner upset, friends may stop making contact or offering support at a time when parents most need it.

Annie's Story

Release is essential, and it may take many months or years before the process is complete. Annie shared her story several months ago at a seminar.

Adequate support was not available at the time of her son's death. Annie was 20 at the time and living on an air force base in New Hampshire.

> *I gave birth to David in 1963 and he lived about two hours. I was in so much pain. I'd lost my first child and I was so drugged. They gave me a saddle block. I had to roll up into a ball, putting my knees on my ears (I can't put my body in this position today.) They told me if I moved the wrong way, I'd be paralyzed for life. Then more drugs. Somehow I heard them talking about how they could set up a spot to give the news to my dad. They were afraid dad would have a heart attack. I thought I was dead myself and somehow could still hear.*
>
> *I asked about the baby. I wanted to know what was happening but I was so drugged I couldn't scream. My husband was away in the service and I felt like I had no one. The doctor told me David had died. He was a Down's Syndrome child. The doctor said that I should be glad he died because he would never have been right. I said, "Okay." I was frozen. I should have screamed, but I couldn't. Later I walked down to the nursery to see my girlfriend's baby. The nurses went berserk. I said I was going to look at the baby and they grabbed me and pushed me back into my room. They said there was no baby. I meant my girlfriend's baby. I really needed to hold someone's baby.*
>
> *My mom called to find out when I could come home and the nurse told her that the doctor was thinking of transferring me to the state mental hospital. My parents stood by me. They knew I wasn't crazy.*
>
> *My husband got home and the doctor convinced him I needed to be institutionalized, and he agreed to support the doctor. My mom stood by me. I went home and my husband and I were never okay again. Five years later we got divorced.*
>
> *Since David's death, I have seen films on Down's Syndrome children. The children are difficult at times but beautiful children. They were warm, loving, with so much to give. How could anyone tell me I was lucky my son died? It took me nineteen years to let that go.*

Healing

In Chapter Ten, grieving is described as a holistic process involving the recovery of the body, mind, heart, and soul. Understanding what is happening relaxes the mind and eases added fears of being "crazy" or inappropriate. There are several excellent materials providing an in-depth view of pregnancy loss, that can be recommended for the parent-in-grief: Susan Borg and Judith Lasker's *When Pregnancy Fails* (1981), Larry Peppers and Ronald Knapp's *Motherhood and Mourning* (1980), Hank Pizer and Christine O'Brien Palinski's *Coping with a Miscarriage* (1980), Harriet Sarnoff Schiff's *The Bereaved Parent* (1977), and my own *Ended Beginnings* (forthcoming).

In addition to reading, the sharing of one's experience is also essential.

Often, sharing with parents who have experienced a similar loss is very consoling and relieving. Support groups such as AMEND (Aiding a Mother Experiencing Neonatal Death), HOPE (Helping Other Parents Endure), and Compassionate Friends* are very helpful when grieving parents, especially women, still need to share, cry, and find hope. Family and friends may tire of listening, and grieving parents require ongoing support for their stories and feelings, which may need to be expressed a thousand times.

The following guidelines are offered to assist in the grieving process as concepts conducive not only to grieving but also to a renewed lifestyle. There are times that grief, depression, and despair may block our ability to understand that fetal and infant death impact profoundly on our lives. It would be impossible to ever be the same. Some may use this time to mourn, to grieve, and to find a deeper sense of understanding and awareness.

Guidelines for Grieving

1. BE A SUPPORTABLE PERSON

Cast your pride to the wind and allow others to know who you really are and what is truly happening! Withholding and trying to "be strong" prolongs grief, deepens our sorrow, alienates our hearts. Suffering in silence is not helpful. This doesn't mean you won't want to grieve alone from time to time.

2. FIND SUPPORT

Cast your pride to the wind and find unconditional supporters, who will love and listen until you are tired of talking or crying or yelling. Advice is rarely useful. No one can give you back your baby but some may help you heal.

3. MAKE KNOWN YOUR NEEDS

Cast your pride to the wind and be specific about what you want and need. If you need company, ask for it. If you don't want it, ask your company to leave. People need to know how to help and support. No one will guess right.

4. ASK QUESTIONS

Cast your pride to the wind. Ask questions. Every unanswered question is a potential guilt. Ask your questions many times. Ask many people.

---

*A list of support groups and their addresses appears after the Bibliography.

Don't stop until you are satisfied that you can go no further. You deserve the best answers medicine has to offer. Foggy, unclear answers are unacceptable. Keep asking if you need to.

5. LOVE, HONOR, AND RESPECT YOUR BODY

Cast your pride to the wind. Your body is vulnerable to illness and pain. It needs good food. It needs extra rest. It needs relaxation. Get touched. Don't have sex until you are ready. Tell others how to care for your body. Without adequate touch, nutrition, and rest, recovery time will be severely prolonged.

6. RESOLVE YOUR RELATIONSHIPS

Cast your pride to the wind. If others offend you, tell them. Teach them how to grieve. Teach them what to say. End relationships you are done with on a peaceful note. This will be a time of emotional house-cleaning. Good friendships will become deeper. Don't hold grudges. They hurt too much, and you are already hurt enough. Little hurts easily become mountainous unless shared. Try not to write off your friends for saying stupid things or because they seem insensitive. We've all done our share of unconscious hurting of others.

7. LOVE YOUR CHILD FOREVER, OPENLY

Cast your pride to the wind. Talk about your child whenever you feel like it (within supportive contexts). Don't try to forget anything you don't feel like forgetting. Leave baby pictures, foot-prints, hair, toys, any reminders out to view if you so desire. Never let anyone talk you into thinking your relationship with your child is pathological.

A Visualization Process

The following is a guided imagery based on a dream-work process developed by psychologist Jack Johnston (1978) out of his studies of the Senoi culture's use of dream-life for creative works and psychological healing. Beginning with a relaxation process, the parents are given (or give themselves) the following suggestions:

> *Now that your body and mind are peaceful and calm, allow yourself to drift off to some place in the world that you feel would support a meeting once again between you and your child. You may have visited this place*

many times or perhaps you've never been here before. Take your time and locate yourself in a place that will truly honor this meeting. Good. Breathe and relax.

Now imagine that you are surrounding this place with complete support and protection. Perhaps the protection may be built in the form of energy—white healing light—or with good friends who know their place of support and do not intrude on this private time, or, for some, perhaps you'll choose guardian angels or spirits who may already seem to be protecting your child. Good. Breathe and relax. Let go on the out breath. Good.

When you feel ready, look off into the distance and see your child in some physical form. This is a meeting beyond the body, of love, and of the essence of each person. You may see your son or daughter as an infant who floats on a cloud or a young child of 6 or 8 or 10. Whatever physical image you envision, remember that it is a meeting of one essence to another. Allow the image to come closer, close enough so that you are able to communicate with one another in comfort. Good. Breathe.

If you feel tears, welcome them—for tears are the rivers of life that cleanse the heart and soul. They are signs of sorrow but also of love. Remember, you are completely safe in this space to cry and let go—to breathe and let go.

Now, will you give your child the power to communicate in a way that you will be sure to understand. The essence of soul is always to communicate, regardless of whether he or she has use of language. Good.

Gazing at your child, I'd like you to ask your son or daughter if there is anything he or she wants from you, anything he or she might need in order to be at peace. Allow all the time you need. The answer will be given, so try to allow yourself to be open to what will now come to you. If your child tells you that he or she is in need of something, take the time now to provide for your child. Remember, in this space everything is possible and all wishes can be granted. Good. Breathe.

Once you have given your child what is needed, ask for a gift—not just any gift, but rather for what might be called an essence gift. An essence gift is like the best possible present one can give another, a present that may symbolize a deeper meaning. Open your heart to receive this gift. Allow the gift to come from your child, even though you may not understand it. Good. Breathe and accept what is given.

Take the gift into your possession—keep it always as a sign of this permanent and indestructible bond that no one can interrupt. Take a few minutes to thank your child, as he or she thanks you for this time together.

Now it is time to begin to slowly leave this place. But before you do, allow your child to drift away just as he or she appeared, remembering that you may visit him or her at any time on this plane. Allow yourself to also take in this place. Notice now that you may go here any time you need to—just to visit or to share.

Bring with you the gift you received. See that gift as a symbol and receive from it new strength. Slowly come back into the room. Gently notice the sounds, the feelings of your chair or the floor. Slowly bring yourself back.

Before you are completely back, make a commitment to get for yourself some actual, physical manifestation of what you've received. It needn't be an exact replica but a symbol that feels just right—trust yourself to know when you have it.

Amy's Story

The following account demonstrates the use of this particular visualization for a couple who found great healing in the process.

Amy lost her daughter, Tara, two hours after birth. Amy had carried to full term and seemed to have a normal pregnancy. Tara was delivered vaginally after a seven-hour labor. The delivery was very pleasing to Amy, since her son had been delivered by Cesarean section.

Tara had multiple birth defects, including a malformed lower-intestinal septum. Joe, Amy's husband, immediately said that he wanted to hold Tara, and encouraged Amy to do the same.

In an act of absolute courage, Amy and Joe named their daughter, held her, and said good-bye to her. They did so against the advice of medical personnel, and they felt they had to fight to claim their child.

After several months of grieving, they came to us because they felt a deep lack of peace and a painful hole in their lives. They both wanted children, yet felt they could not become pregnant again until they resolved their loss.

We recalled the events of the pregnancy and birth and settled these so that both Amy and Joe could move on to full grieving of Tara. Then, we introduced the healing process derived from the Senoi ritual.

We asked them each, in separate sessions, to see Tara as they remembered her, focusing her into view as best they could, and to let us know when they saw her. We then asked them to ask Tara from their hearts—not minds—if she wanted anything further. Amy said Tara wanted her, Amy, to forgive herself. Joe said Tara wanted nothing.

We asked Amy if she would be willing to forgive herself. Amy replied that she would. We then asked each of them to ask Tara to take them to the source of her power. Tara took each of them (without their consulting with each other) to the summer home where she had been conceived.

We then invited Amy and Joe, separately, to ask Tara for a gift—a gift that would represent her appreciation toward them as loving parents and a sign of their eternal love. Each of them received a heart. Amy's came in the form of a gold locket. Joe's came in the form of a red valentine. (As far as we know, neither consulted the other before doing the process.)

We then invited each of them to go out into the world and find these gifts, to bring them home, and to keep them as reminders of Tara and the eternal love between them.

We then asked each of them to let Tara know that they would be okay—so that if she, Tara, needed to move on anywhere, she would be free to do so. We reminded Amy and Joe that they would never forget or stop loving Tara, and added that if anyone ever encouraged them to do so, to reject this advice immediately. However, loving a child and suffering were very different, and we asked them to consider never suffering unneccessarily again—to welcome their sorrow and tears but never to suffer from self-criticism, or attempts at justifying, or anything else.

Last year Amy and Joe gave birth to a beautiful son, Matthew. They brought Tara's gifts to Matthew's birth and felt they acquired much self-confidence from her symbolic presence. They grieved and healed and allowed the birds of sorrow to pass without nesting in their hair.

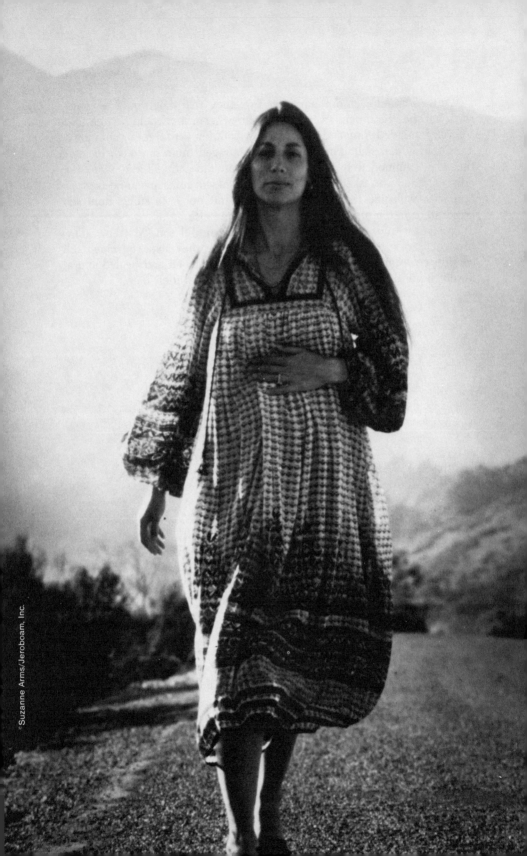

13

Childbirth in the Aquarian Age

It is said that we are entering the Age of Aquarius, a time of enlightenment and change through community effort. We are leaving an age of individual gain, of competition, and of the self-centered, ego-building consciousness; and moving to a time when accomplishment, creativity, and intuition are to be directed toward the betterment of the human condition.

Today, many environmental, political, and social groups are working for constructive change, perhaps evidence that great transformation has begun. Marilyn Ferguson wrote, in *The Aquarian Conspiracy* (1980), "Broader than reform, deeper than revolution, this benign conspiracy for a new human agenda has triggered the most rapid cultural realignment in history." She was speaking to the mandate for change needed in our institutions and systems. This mandate has not escaped the field of childbirth, childbearing parents, or the obstetrical community at large.

Change: The Efforts of Many

The movement began slowly in the 1940s and 1950s with the work of Dr. Fernand Lamaze and Dr. Grantly Dick-Read, who first brought natural childbirth to the United States. Dick-Read directed his energies toward neutralizing maternal fears, while Lamaze developed breathing and exercise techniques for childbearing women. Their work, and that of Robert Bradley,

171

opened our eyes to the importance of emotional support and to the idea of father involvement in the birthing process.

In the 1960s Sheila Kitzinger wrote *The Experience of Childbirth* (1981). As a researcher, mother, and noted anthropologist, Kitzinger spoke of the significance of the emotional aspects of birth and the need for parents to understand this process in order to produce genuine joy in childbirth. Ms. Kitzinger's work was significant not only because she underlined the emotional aspects of childbearing and promoted surrender to the body over disciplined breathing, but also because she was a woman speaking to women.

Then began over a decade of works that challenged and questioned obstetrical practice and procedure. Doris Haire (1972) compiled a special report to the International Childbirth Education Association, in which she questioned many standard policies and documented the innate risks in many of our standard procedures today. Suzanne Arms came forth with her blatantly confronting material *Immaculate Deception* (1975), further uncovering the myths and madness inherent in American obstetrics. Ina May Gaskin, in *Spiritual Midwifery* (1977), validated midwifery and shared her birthing success at "the Farm," an alternative community in Tennessee.

The famous Frederick Leboyer (1976) taught us to birth gently and recognized the newborn's right to respectful treatment while the Hathaways wrote *Children at Birth* (1978) because they understood the psychological impact of birth and the personal needs and feelings of siblings as family members.

David and Lee Stewart formed NAPSAC (National Alliance of Parents and Professionals for Safe Alternatives in Childbirth), an organization that has promoted change in unsafe obstetrical practices. Other groups—such as SPUN (Society for the Protection of the Unborn through Nutrition), founded on the work of Tom and Gail Brewer; the home birth movement, aided by the supportive documentation of Lewis Mehl; and the Cesarean Prevention Movement, led by women such as Nancy Cohen, coauthor of *Silent Knife* (Cohen & Estner 1983)—have all responded to the Aquarian Age mandate for human betterment in obstetrical care.

There are many others whose efforts have brought about a new consciousness on the state of obstetrics and a new awareness of the psychological needs of childbearing parents. There are birthing rooms and alternative centers developing throughout the land. The movement to return childbirth to women, to supportive environments, and to healthy expression of normal human functioning rather than a medical emergency, has a momentum that will not yield in spite of setbacks and opposition.

In these times of change and challenge, it is difficult to know what is right and responsible. The misuse of Cesarean deliveries, of drugs, of other medical technologies is under question. The consumer is challenged to become informed of it all.

The Challenged Consumer

The transition from the treatment of pregnancy and birth as disease to the acceptance of childbearing as healthy and normal is in process. The role of the father is expanding. The return of the midwife to her rightful role is creating political obstetrics while most childbearing parents are working hard to do what is right for themselves and their children.

Childbearing parents are more vulnerable than ever to feelings of guilt, failure, and inadequacy. We can read volumes of material, attend the best possible childbirth education courses, and become totally healthy through correct diet and proper exercise. We can examine our beliefs, think positive thoughts, and practice visualizations. We can lay out a birth plan that calls for maximum support and minimal intervention, find the best possible physician or midwife, and completely prepare our children for birth. In fact, we owe it to ourselves to exert all of these conscious efforts.

"Angels Can Do No Better"

However, we also owe it to ourselves to remain aware that no matter what the outcome or events, we as parents have simply done our best. The kindly encouragement of my first-grade teacher who once told our class, "Do your best; angels can do no better," is true for us as adults today. In the final analysis, that is all we can expect of ourselves. It is hardly likely that a woman who is surgically delivered planned the delivery in order to take "the easy way out." Any Cesarean mother can tell you that surgical birth is far from easy. It is unlikely that any couple who prepare for natural childbirth plan for medical interventions, drugs, and difficult births. It is painfully shocking to expect and plan for a healthy baby and give birth to an injured or stillborn child. None of us consciously wants distress and disappointment.

Although it is true that we are ultimately responsible for all of the events in our lives, including pregnancy and childbirth, it is cruel to continuously ask ourselves why we "made" ourselves have a miscarriage, a Cesarean, or a medicated birth. The "why" cannot heal the hurt incurred, nor can it alter the future.

It is, however, critical that we remain conscious of how we feel about our childbearing experiences and how we hold the emotions of these events within our hearts. There may be a fine line between consciousness and self-criticism, but our feelings are a clear guide to knowing when we have crossed it.

Responsibility—Not Guilt

The fundamental aim of this work is to increase one's conscious awareness of feelings and to better understand how to healthily integrate *all* life events, regardless of outcome. Childbirth is a time of great learning and emotional growth. Hopefully, it will be used as such.

Although it is our belief that the mind influences the body, it is also our knowledge that no human being can ever expect to fully know all the thoughts and beliefs in that mind. Further, it has become increasingly evident in our work with the childbearing process that our life on this planet is not without purpose. Each of us seems to be here with a specific task, a series of important life lessons, and a "soul" path, perhaps beyond our own comprehension. For some of us, unraveling the events of our childbirth experiences will be the arena for those life learnings and maybe even the guide to our soul's path. In order for this learning to take place, we may need the consciousness and even the conflict of the childbearing process.

Members of Alcoholics Anonymous believe that God only gives us what we are able to handle and what we need in order to grow. Some of us may need the difficulties and emotional hurts of our childbirth experiences in order for growth to take place.

It seems increasingly clear to us that parents who have the consciousness to use childbearing as a growth opportunity seem to gain in personal strength, resources, and depth of relationship. They often alter many other areas of their lives, such as their relationships with their own parents, children, and friends, as a result of their learning through emotionally conscious childbearing. These parents exhibit great emotional resources, strength, and health.

Awakening the Feeling of Consciousness

We believe that it may be difficult for many parents to allow full consciousness of their feelings and thoughts when Western psychotherapeutic traditions tend to offer an instant pathological diagnosis for those who do allow awareness and expression of feelings. Just as we are attempting to return the treatment of the physiology of childbirth to the philosophy of birth as a healthy condition rather than an impending disease, so, too, are we, in this work, attempting to approach the expression of feelings and thoughts as natural, healthy, nonpathological consciousness worthy of support, not diagnosis. This approach to childbirth may assist parents in truly acknowledging whatever is going on inside of them regardless of whether it seems rational and appropriate or not.

Each of us has the responsibility to become an informed consumer. Geoffrey Hodson (1981) wrote:

> The duty and responsibility of all who undertake the office of parenthood is therefore very heavy. Pure, sensitive, refined and healthy bodies are needed for the advanced egos who are to lead and guide humanity in the building of a new civilization. . . . The parents of the children of the new

age must be inspired by the highest spiritual ideals and must recognize that man's [*sic*] power to create is a divine attribute.

Yes, we must be so inspired. We have an equally important responsibility to ourselves. We owe ourselves, above all else, peace of mind.

The material in this book has been offered to assist parents and professionals in further understanding birth as a psychophysiological process. It is offered to support healthy and positive psychological integration of all pregnancy and childbirth experiences. It is hoped that readers will use this material to achieve greater peace of mind through such integration and through self-acceptance.

The Ultimate Task: Self-Acceptance

Each of us is given the task of self-acceptance. Some of us are given very difficult circumstances in which to find it. The childbearing years offer much challenge to our psychological self-evaluation systems. For the woman who has had an abortion, her task is not to suffer for her decision. Women do not abort because they hate children. In fact, they usually do so because they feel unable to bring a child into their lives at this time.

For the woman who has delivered surgically, her task is to see that she was attempting to save her baby's life through an act of personal courage. The surgery is violating enough, without a lifetime of guilt to follow. Forgiveness and self-acceptance are the path to peace of mind.

For the medicated mother and her (sometimes unnecessarily) monitored child, her task is to recognize the lifetime of medical orientation that is not easily altered—an orientation that has led all of us to believe the myth that drugs and machines always save lives and do no potential harm.

For all birthing parents whose dreams did not come true, there is enough suffering in a lost dream, without a lifetime of recriminations.

It is difficult for any of us to find forgiveness for ourselves and others when we are hurt. Yet, without forgiveness, we suffer permanently. In these times of obstetrical change and consumer challenge of past practices, emotional issues are often further complicated. However, without forgiveness for all, we shall never be granted peace of mind.

Life Lessons of Childbirth

Denise and Stewart's Story

Denise and Stewart's story reminds us of how much is asked of each of us and how far down inside ourselves we must sometimes reach in order to forgive.

Their story involves some of the painful political events in the practice of obstetrics today and speaks to the profoundly difficult task of self-forgiveness and self-acceptance each of us must undertake within our own life circumstances.

On Friday, Denise's midwife requested a non-stress test because Denise was some two weeks past her due date and was planning a home birth. Denise and her husband Stewart went to the hospital for the test and met the physician's associate covering for their chosen doctor while he vacationed.

Denise was frightened at the prospect of entering a hospital even for tests, since she knew that interventions carried risks and wanted as few as possible. The non-stress test results indicated some possible difficulty, although not absolute. The covering physician, hurried by his overwhelming schedule, encouraged the couple to remain in the hospital and to allow induction.

Horrified at the thought of hospital deliveries and disturbed at the shattering of the dreams of ideal home birthing, Denise and Stewart asked for a few moments of discussion and some time to make such a decision. The physician ordered a second test. A second non-stress test was given and the results indicated no problem.

Denise and Stewart decided to go home for the weekend and to return on Monday if labor had not begun. Given the results of the more supportive second test and several recent studies on postmaturity, the physician again supported their decision. Denise and Stewart went home for the weekend, promising to return on Monday if labor had not begun by then.

The next day labor started spontaneously. Like most of the pregnancy, the labor went well, contractions increased, and Denise dilated to some 7 centimeters. Suddenly, the attending midwife announced she could not get a fetal heartbeat. After several tries, they transferred to the nearby hospital and called the physician. Efforts were unsuccessful and their baby died. No one knew why, and Denise was left with the horror of continuing labor, knowing she would give birth to a lifeless child. Denise and Stewart were very well informed. They had attended private childbirth-preparation courses and knew well the risks and advantages of home birthing. They ate well and did everything possible to birth normally and to prepare for a healthy child.

Because of their knowledge of the innate risks in medical intervention and their desire to begin family life in their own home, they chose not to enter a hospital. Their birth experience, and others like theirs, have become the target of much debate.

The Pain of Critical Judgment

Fortunately or unfortunately, whenever there is change, there is always resistance to change. There are those who oppose home birth and wave the finger of "I told you so," a sad and wholly inappropriate note, because *no one will ever know* if Joshua (or any child in that position) could have survived labor, would have been saved by a Cesarean, or would have been further compromised by an induced labor. No one knows whether the greatest technological advances in the world would have saved Joshua, and to proclaim some ability to know an alternate future creates unnecessary suffering to already burdened parents.

Robert Mendelsohn, M.D., Nancy Cohen, Gena Corea, Lewis Mehl, and other Aquarian conspirators are working to unravel the truth of modern obstetrics and to create a new worldview of the childbirth experience. Others seek to hold on to the more traditional approaches of hospital birthing, including procedural drugs, episiotomies, and ever-higher rates of Cesarean delivery. Perhaps one day the hospital will evolve into a safe place to seek emergency medical intervention, with absolute respect for childbearing women. Perhaps one day all alternatives for childbirth will be the welcoming, emotionally supportive environments we all naturally desire. Until that day, childbearing Western men and women must find self-acceptance in the knowledge that they have done their best.

" . . .And the Walls Came Tumbling Down!"

Autopsy results showed no specific cause for Joshua's death. Whether Joshua would have died under other circumstances is known only to God herself. Stewart and Denise live every day with the loss of their son, hopefully feeling every moment that they did what they believed was right and that "angels could do no better."

The Age of Aquarius calls for hope in a better future. Marilyn Ferguson (1980) calls it "a movement into the unknown because the known has failed us too completely." Childbirth in the Aquarian Age begins with group effort and group support of each individual parent. It calls for change in obstetrical practices and attempts at unknown possibilities and alternatives. It calls for communicating and linking our efforts, so that no one suffers unnecessarily as a result of the movement, and for confronting our own individual responsibility to take part in effecting change.

To this point, Marilyn Ferguson quotes a Robert Frost poem: "Something we were withholding made us weak, until we found it was ourselves." Let us not withhold either our individual feelings that need release or our group efforts that need action and implementation.

Denise and Stewart named their son Joshua because of a special, spiritual meaning he has in their lives. Joshua of Biblical fame was a leader of his people. He set forth to battle what he believed needed change. In the end, he built an altar as a witness to God, uniting two groups separated by the Jordan River, two groups that were not yet united in service. Perhaps one day the Jericho walls of modern obstetrical policy and standard procedure will come tumbling down and our daughters and sons will know the peace of a bridge built across the Jordan River when all groups unite for positive, conscious birthing. Until then, let us not deny ourselves our own peace of mind. We owe it to ourselves and to those who rely on us.

Support Groups

AMEND (Aiding a Mother Experiencing Neonatal Death)
 Los Angeles Chapter
 4032 Towhee Drive
 Calabassas, Calif. 91302

HOPE (Help Other Parents Endure)
 c/o Susan Harrington
 South Shore Hospital
 55 Fogg Road
 South Weymouth, Mass. 02190
 (617) 337-7011, ext. 332

The Compassionate Friends, Inc.
 P.O. Box 1347
 Oak Brook, Ill. 60521
 (313) 323-5010

Loving Relationships Training, a 3-day workshop created by Dondra Ray.
 18321 Ventura Blvd., Suite 1010
 Tarzana, Calif. 91350

Bibliography & References

Adams, Margaret E., & Joyce Prince. 1978. *Minds, Mothers and Midwives*. New York: Longman.

Allen, Brian. 1972. "Liberating the Manchild." *Transactional Analysis Journal*, 2:68–71.

American College of Obstetricians and Gynecologists. 1982. "Maternal and Fetal Medicine Guidelines for Vaginal Birth after Cesarean Childbirth." Available from ACOG, 600 Maryland Ave., S.W., Suite 300 E, Washington, D.C. 20024.

Arms, Suzanne. 1977. *Immaculate Deception*. New York: Bantam Books.

Asch, S., & L. Rubin. 1974. "Postpartum Reactions: Some Unrecognized Variations." *American Journal of Psychiatry*, 131:8.

Bandler, Richard, & John Grinder. 1975, 1976. *The Structure of Magic*, 2 vols. Palo Alto, Cal.: Science and Behavior Books.

Bean, Constance. 1970. *Labor and Delivery: An Observer's Diary*. Garden City, N.Y.: Doubleday.

Berne, Eric. 1972. *What Do You Say after You Say Hello?* New York: Grove.

Bibring, G., et al. 1961. "A Study of the Earliest Mother-Child Relationship." *Psychoanalytic Study of the Child*, 16, no. 9.

Birnbaum, S.J., R.G. Douglas, & F.A. MacDonald. 1963. "Pregnancies and Labor Following Cesarean Section." *American Journal of Obstetrics and Gynecology*, 86 (Aug.).

Bittman, Sam, & Sue Rosenberg Zalk. 1978. *Expectant Fathers*. New York: Ballantine Books.

Black, Jean L., & Deborah Tanzer. 1972. *Why Natural Childbirth?* Garden City, N.Y.: Doubleday.

Borg, Susan, & Judith Lasker. 1981. *When Pregnancy Fails*. Boston: Beacon.

Boston Women's Health Book Collective. 1978. *Ourselves and Our Children*. New York: Random House.

Brackbill, Yvonne, M.D., J. Kane, R.L. Maniello, M.D., & D. Abramson, M.D. 1974. "Fetus, Placenta and Newborn: Obstetric Premedication and Infant Outcome." *American Journal of Obstetrics and Gynecology,* 118:337–83.

Bradley, Robert. 1965. *Husband Coached Childbirth.* New York: Harper & Row.

Brazelton, T. Berry, M.D. 1979. *Doctor and Child.* New York: Delta Books, Dell. 1981   *On Becoming a Family.* New York: Delacorte.

Brennan, Barbara, & Joan Rattner Heilman. 1977. *The Complete Book of Midwifery.* New York: E. P. Dutton.

Brewer, Gail Sforza. 1977. *What Every Pregnant Woman Should Know.* New York: Penguin.

Brewer, Gail Sforza, & Janice Presser Greene. 1981. *Right from the Start.* Emmaus, Pa.: Rodale.

Bromberg, Joann. 1981. "Having a Baby: A Story Essay." *Childbirth: Alternatives to Medical Control.* Austin: University of Texas Press.

Browne, Alan, & James McGrath. 1965. "Vaginal Delivery after Previous Cesarean Section." *Obstetrics-Gynecology of the British Commonwealth,* 72:557.

Brown-Hill, Barbara, & Lynn Baptisti Richards. Forthcoming. *The Vaginal Birth after Cesarean Workbook.* South Hadley, Mass.: Bergin & Garvey.

Bry, Adelaide. 1979. *Visualization: Directing the Movies of Your Mind.* New York: Harper & Row.

Bureau of Natality, Statistics Department. 1981. *1980 Statistics.* Vital Records, Rm. 100, 615 Penn. Ave., N.W., Washington, D.C. 20004.

Cohen, Nancy. 1977. "Minimizing the Emotional Sequellae of Cesarean Birth." *Birth and the Family Journal,* Fall.

Cohen, Nancy, & Lois Estner. 1983. *Silent Knife: Cesarean Prevention and Vaginal Birth after Cesarean.* South Hadley, Mass.: Bergin & Garvey.

Colen, B.D. 1981. *Born at Risk.* New York: St. Martin's.

Corea, Gena. 1978. *The Hidden Malpractice.* New York: Harcourt Brace Jovanovich.

Cousins, Norman. 1979. *The Anatomy of an Illness as Told by the Patient.* Toronto, Canada: N.W. Norton.

Creighton, T., O.C. Simonton, & S. Matthews-Simonton. 1978. *Getting Well Again.* Los Angeles: Tarcher.

de Jim, Strange. 1979. *Visioning.* San Francisco: Ash-Kar.

Delliquadri, Lyn, & Kati Breckenridge. 1979. *MotherCare.* New York: Pocket Books.

Deutsch, Helene. 1945. *The Psychology of Women,* vol. 2. New York: Bantam Books.

Diamond, John. 1980. *The Collected Papers of John Diamond, M.D.,* vol. 2. Valley Cottage, N.Y.: Archaeus.

Dick-Read, Grantly. 1944. *Childbirth without Fear.* New York: Harper & Row.

Dinkmeyer, Don, & Lewis E. Losconcy. 1980. *The Encouragement Book.* Englewood Cliffs, N.J.: Prentice-Hall.

Douglas, R.G., S.J. Birnbaum, & F.A. MacDonald. 1963. "Pregnancy and Labor following Cesarean Section." *American Journal of Obstetrics and Gynecology,* 86:9–61.

Dowling, Colette. 1980. *The Cinderella Complex.* New York: Pocket Books.

Duncan, Judith. 1982. "Preparation for Parenthood: A Case for Prevention." Paper presented at the Perinatal Social Workers' Conference, Houston, Texas, 28 May.

Emery, Stewart. 1978. *Actualizations: You Don't Have to Rehearse to Be Yourself.* Garden City, N.Y.: Dolphin Books.

Fein, R.A. 1976. "Men's Entrance to Parenthood." *Family Coordinator*, 254:341–48.

Feldman, Silvia. 1978. *Choices in Childbirth.* New York: Grosset & Dunlap.

Fraiberg, Selma. 1977. *Every Child's Birthright: In Defense of Mothering.* New York: Basic Books.

Freud, Sigmund. 1932. *Concerning the Sexuality of Women."* *Psychoanalytic Quarterly*, 1.

Friday, Nancy. 1978. *My Mother, My Self.* New York: Dell.

Friedman, Rochelle, M.D., & Bonnie Gradstein. 1982. *Surviving Pregnancy Loss.* Boston: Little, Brown.

Gaskin, Ina May. 1977. *Spiritual Midwifery.* Summertown, Tenn.: Book Pub.

Gawain, Shakti. 1978. *Creative Visualization.* Mill Valley, Cal. Whatever Pub.

Gordon, Tom. 1974. *Parent Effectiveness Training.* New York: Peter H. Wyden.

Gots, Barbara, & Ronald Gots. 1977. *Caring for Your Unborn Child.* New York: Bantam Books.

Grollman, Earl. 1981. *What Helped Me When My Loved One Died.* Boston: Beacon.

Guttmacher, Alan F., M.D. 1973. *Pregnancy, Birth, and Family Planning.* New York: Viking (orig. pub. 1937).

Haire, Doris. 1972. *The Cultural Warping of Childbirth.* Hillside, N.J.: ICEA.

1981 *Research in Drugs Used in Pregnancy and Obstetrics.* Washington, D.C.: Subcommittee on Investigation and Oversight of the House Committee on Science and Technology.

Hamburg, D.A., D.T. Lunde, R.H. Moss, & I.D. Yalom. 1968. "Postpartum Blues Syndrome." *Archives of Genetic Psychiatry*, 18:16–27.

Harlow, H.F., & M.K. Harlow. 1966. "Learning to Love." *American Scientist*, 54:244–72.

Harrison, Mary. 1979. *Infertility: A Guide for Couples.* Boston: Houghton Mifflin.

Harrison, Michelle, M.D. 1982. *A Woman in Residence.* New York: Random House.

Hathaway, Jay, & Marjie Hathaway. 1978. *Children at Birth.* Sherman Oaks, Cal.: Academy.

Hazell, Lester. 1976. *Commonsense Childbirth*, rev. 2d ed. New York: Berkley.

Hodson, Geoffrey. 1981. *The Miracle of Birth.* Wheaton, Ill.: Theosophical Pub. House.

Hovey, Wendy Roe, & Christine Coleman Wilson. 1980. *Cesarean Childbirth.* Garden City, N.Y.: Dolphin Books.

Howe, Leland W., Howard Kirschenbaum, & Sidney B. Simon. 1978. *Values Clarification*, rev. ed. New York: A & W Pub.

James, Muriel, & Dorothy Jongeward. 1973. *Born to Win.* Reading, Mass.: Addison-Wesley.

James, William. 1950. *The Principles of Psychology.* U.S.A.: Dover.

Jameson, Beth. 1971. *Hold Me Tight.* Old Tappan, N.J.: Fleming H. Revell.

Jampolsky, Gerald G. 1979. *Love Is Letting Go of Fear.* Millbrae, Cal.: Celestial Arts.

Janov, Arthur. 1971. *The Anatomy of Mental Illness.* New York: G.P. Putnum's Sons.

Jensen, Joseph & Rothlyn Zahourek. 1972. "Depression in Mothers Who Have Lost a Newborn." *Rocky Mountain Medical Journal,* 69:61–63.

Johnston, Jack. 1978. "Senoi Dreamwork." *Sundance Community Dream Journal,* 2 (Winter): 50–61.

Jones, Terry. 1980a. *Also of Men Born! Chapter 3: Father the Heavy.* West Linn, Ore.: Also of Men Born Series.

   1980b   *Also of Men Born! Chapter 5: The Experience of Pregnancy.* West Linn, Ore.: Also of Men Born Series.

Jongeward, Dorothy, & Dru Scott. 1976. *Women as Winners.* Reading, Mass.: Addison-Wesley.

Jordan, Brigitte. 1980. *Birth in Four Cultures.* Montreal: Eden Press Women's Pub.

Kagan, J., H.A. Moss, & I.F. Siegel. 1963. "The Psychological Significance of Styles of Conceptualization," in *Basic Cognitive Processes in Children,* ed. J.C. Wright & J. Kagan. Monographs of the Society for Research in Child Development, vol. 28, no. 2.

Kenefick, Madeleine. 1981. *Positively Pregnant.* Los Angeles: Pinnacle Books.

Keyes, Ken, Jr. 1979. *A Conscious Person's Guide to Relationships.* St. Mary, Kan.: Living Love.

Kirk, Paul, & Pat Schwiebert. 1981. *When Hello Means Goodbye.* Portland: University of Oregon Health Science Center.

Kitzinger, Sheila. 1980. *The Complete Book of Pregnancy and Childbirth.* New York: Alfred Knopf.

   1981   *The Experience of Childbirth,* 4th ed. New York: Pelican/Penguin Books.

Klaus, Marshall H., & John H. Kennell. 1980. *Parent-Infant Bonding.* St. Louis, Mo.: C.V. Mosby Co.

Kubler-Ross, Elisabeth. 1969. *On Death and Dying.* New York: Macmillan.

   1974   *Questions and Answers on Death and Dying.* New York: Macmillan.

Lamaze, Fernand. 1958. *Painless Childbirth.* New York: Pocket Books.

Leboyer, Frederick. 1974. *Birth without Violence.* London: Wildwood House.

   1975   "Birth without Violence: An Evening with F. Leboyer." *Journal of Primal Therapy,* 2:295.

   1976   *Loving Hands.* New York: Alfred A. Knopf.

Lewis, Emmanuel. 1976. "The Management of Stillbirth: Coping with an Unreality." *Lancet,* 2:619–20.

Lowen, Alexander. 1972. *Depression and the Body.* Baltimore: Penguin Books.

   1975   *Bioenergetics.* New York: Penguin Books.

Marieskind, Helen. 1979. *An Evaluation of Cesarean Section in the United States: A Report to the Department of Health, Education and Welfare.* Washington, D.C.: HEW.

Mathison, Linda. 1980. "Down the Tunnel: An Inquiry into the Memories of the Very Young." *Federal Monitor,* 3 (28 Nov.).

Mehl, Lewis, M.D. 1978. "Home Delivery Research Today: A Review," in *A Place of Birth,* ed. S. Kitzenger. Oxford University Press.

1979 "The Importance of Belief in the Childbearing Process," in *Five Standards for Safe Childbirth*, eds. L. and D. Stewart. Marble Hill, MO: KNAPSAC.

Mehl, Lewis, & Gail Peterson. 1979. "The Role of Some Birth-Related Variables and Father Attachment." *American Journal of Orthopsychiatry*, 49:330–38.

Meltzer, David. 1981. *Birth*. San Francisco: North Point.

Mendelsohn, Robert S. 1979. *The Confessions of a Medical Heretic*. Chicago: Contemporary Books.

1981 *Mal(e) Practice: How Doctors Manipulate Women*. Chicago: Contemporary Books.

Meyer, Linda D. 1979. *The Cesarean (R) Evolution: A Handbook for Parents and Childbirth Educators*. Edmonds, Wash.: Chas. Franklin.

Montague, Ashley. 1964. *Life before Birth*. New York: New American Library.

Morningstar, Jim. 1980. *Spiritual Psychology*. Available from the author, 2728 Prospect Ave. Milwaukee, Wis. 53211.

Murphy, Joseph. 1963. *The Power of Your Subconscious Mind*. Englewood Cliffs, N.J.: Prentice Hall.

Orr, Leonard. 1977. *Rebirthing in the New Age*. Millbrae, Cal.: Celestial Arts.

Panuthos, Claudia, & Catherine Romeo. Forthcoming. *Ended Beginnings: Healing Pregnancy Losses*. South Hadley, Mass.: Bergin & Garvey.

Pearce, Joseph Chilton. 1977. *Magical Child*. New York: E.P. Dutton.

Peterson, Gayle. 1981. *Birthing Normally*. Berkeley, Cal.: Mindbody.

Peppers, Larry, & Ronald Knapp. 1980. *Motherhood and Mourning: Perinatal Death*. New York: Praeger.

Phillips, Robert D., M.D. 1975. "Structural Symbiotic Systems." Available from the author, 100 Eastowne Dr., Chapel Hill, N.C. 27514.

Pizer, Hank, & C. Palinski. 1980. *Coping with a Miscarriage*. New York: American Library.

Pomeroy, Wardell B. 1981. *Boys and Sex*. New York: Dell.

Ponder, Catherine. 1980. *The Dynamic Laws of Healing*. Marina Del Rey. Cal.: Devorss.

Powell, John. 1973. *Fully Human, Fully Alive*. Niles, Ill.: Argus Communicating.

Rank, Otto. 1929. *The Trauma of Birth*. New York: Harper.

Raphael, Dana. 1973. *The Tender Gift: Breastfeeding*. New York: Schocken Books.

Ray, Sondra. 1976. *I Deserve Love*. Millbrae, Cal.: Les Femmes.

1980 *Loving Relationships*. Millbrae, Cal.: Les Femmes.

Rich, Adrienne. 1976. *Of Woman Born*. New York: Bantam.

Rogers, Carl R. 1961. *On Becoming a Person*. Boston: Houghton Mifflin.

Romalis, Coleman. 1981. "Taking Care of the Little Woman." In S. Romalis et al. 1981.

Romalis, Shelly. 1981. "Natural Childbirth and the Reluctant Physician." In S. Romalis et al. 1981.

Romalis, Shelly, et al., eds. 1981. *Childbirth: Alternatives to Medical Control*. Austin: University of Texas Press.

Rossi, E., & M.H. Erickson. 1974. *Hypnotic Realities*. New York: Irvington.

Samuels, M., and H.Z. Bennett. 1974. *Be Well*. New York: Random House.

Satir, Virginia. 1978. *Your Many Faces*. Millbrae, Cal.: Celestial Arts.

Schiff, Harriet Sarnoff. 1977. *The Bereaved Parent*. New York: Crown.

Sherfan, Andrew Dib. 1971. *Kahlil Gibran: The Nature of Love*. New York: Philosophical Library.

Simonton, Carl, & Stephanie Simonton. 1978. *Getting Well Again*. Los Angeles: Tarcher.

Sousa, Marion. 1976. *Childbirth at Home*. New York: Bantam.

Steiner, Claude. 1974. *Scripts People Live*. New York: Grove.

Stewart, David, & Lee Stewart, eds. 1976. *Safe Alternatives in Childbirth*. Chapel Hill, N.C.: NAPSAC.

Taber, Clarence Wilbur. 1970. *Taber's Cyclopedic Medical Dictionary*. Philadelphia: F.A. Davis.

Trethowan, W.H. 1965. "Expectant Fathers Toothache." *Mother and Child Care*, 1:53.

United States Department of Health and Human Services. 1981. *1981 Statistics*. Rockville, Md.: National Institute of Mental Health.

Vellay, Pierre. 1969. *Childbirth with Confidence*. New York: Macmillan.

Wambach, Helen. 1979. *Life before Life*. New York: Bantam.

Wente, A.S., & S.B. Crockenberg. 1976. "Transition to Fatherhood: Lamaze Preparation Adjustment Difficulty and the Husband-Wife Relationship." *Family Coordinator*, Oct.:351–57.

Williams, Phyllis S. 1974. *Nourishing Your Unborn Child*. New York: Avon.

Willmuth, L.R. 1975. "Prepared Childbirth and the Concept of Control." *Journal of Obstetrical & Gynecological Nursing*, 4(Fall):38.

Wolff, John R. 1970. "The Emotional Reaction to Stillbirth." *American Journal of Obstetrics and Gynecology*, 108:73–77.

Wycoff, Hogie. 1974. "Sex Role Scripting in Men and Woman." In *Scripts People Live*. New York: Grove.

　　1974 "Banal Scripts of Women." In *Scripts People Live*. New York: Grove.

Yalom, I.D., D.T. Lunde, R.H. Moss, & D.A. Hamburg. 1968. "Postpartum Blues Syndrome." *Archives of Genetic Psychiatry*, 18:16–27.

Index

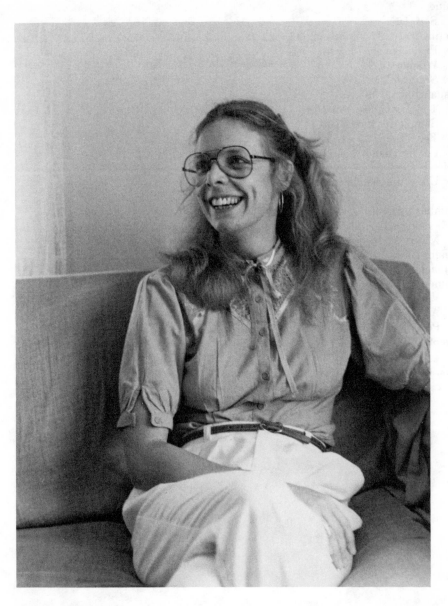

About the Author

CLAUDIA PANUTHOS is founder and director of OFFSPRING, a comprehensive childbirth counseling center. She is the author of many publications, including *Enlightened Parenthood* and *Ended Beginnings* (forthcoming 1984), a national lecturer and consultant, and a frequent guest on TV and radio discussion shows.

Related Books

SILENT KNIFE
Cesarean Prevention
& Vaginal Birth After Cesarean (VBAC)

Nancy Wainer Cohen and Lois J. Estner

Highly acclaimed by all as "an unsurpassed guide to (truly) natural childbirth and the only thorough study of VBAC" *(Library Journal)*; a book that "should be read by every couple contemplating having children" (Ashely Montagu), *Silent Knife* is the first book to expose the scope and severity of the cesarean epidemic—why it has happened, why well-meaning doctors have gotten caught up in it, why it is dangerous—as well as a detailed account, both passionate and level-headed, about what prospective parents can do to *avoid it.*

464 pages/Illustrated/Index
$29.95 Cloth/ISBN 0-89789-026-4
$14.95 Paper/ISBN 0-89789-027-2

Forthcoming Books

ENDED BEGINNINGS
Healing Childbirth Loss

Claudia Panuthos and Catherine Romeo

WOMEN & NUTRITION IN LOW-INCOME COUNTRIES

Barry M. Popkin, Sahni Hamilton, Deborah Spicer